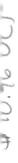

COLOR ATLAS OF SEXUAL ASSAULT

COLOR ATLAS
of
SEXUAL
ASSAULT

BARBARA W. GIRARDIN, RN, PhD
Former Instructor, Graduate Nursing Program
California State University-Dominguez Hills
Dominguez Hills, California
Sexual Assault Nurse Examiner
Palomar-Pomerado Health System
Poway, California

DIANA K. FAUGNO, RN, BSN, CPN, BCFE
Director, Sexual Assault Response Team
Sexual Assault Nurse Examiner
Palomar-Pomerado Health System
Poway, California

PATTY C. SENESKI, RN, ENP
President, International Association of Forensic Nurses
Thorofare, New Jersey
Co-Founder, Sexual Assault Response Team
Sexual Assault Nurse Examiner
Palomar-Pomerado Health System
Poway, California

LAURA SLAUGHTER, MD, FACR, FACP
Former Medical Director
Suspected Abuse Response Team
San Luis Obispo, California

MARGARET WHELAN, RN, BSN
Sexual Assault Nurse Examiner
Palomar-Pomerado Health System
Poway, California

with 221 illustrations

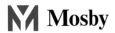 Mosby

St. Louis Baltimore Boston Carlsbad Chicago Minneapolis New York Philadelphia Portland
London Milan Sydney Tokyo Toronto

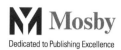
Mosby
Dedicated to Publishing Excellence

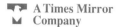
**A Times Mirror
Company**

Vice President and Publisher: Nancy L. Coon
Executive Editor: Sally Schrefer
Associate Developmental Editor: Rae L. Robertson
Project Manager: Deborah L. Vogel
Production Editor: Mamata Reddy
Designer: Pati Pye
Manufacturing Manager: Linda Ierardi

Printed in the United States of America
Composition by TSI Graphics
Printing/binding by Walsworth Printing

Mosby-Year Book, Inc.
11830 Westline Industrial Drive
St. Louis, Missouri 63146

Library of Congress Cataloging in Publication Data
    Color atlas of sexual assault / Barbara W. Girardin ... [et al.].
        p.   cm.
      Includes bibliographical references and index.
      ISBN 0-8151-3842-3 (alk. paper)
       1. Rape victims—Medical examinations—Atlases.   2. Generative organs—Wounds and injuries—
    Atlases. I. Girardin, Barbara W.
      [DNLM: 1. Sex Offenses—atlases.   2. Genitalia—injuries—atlases.   3. Forensic Medicine—methods.
    W617 C719 1997]
    RA1141.C65 1997
    614'.1—dc21
    DNLM/DLC
    for Library of Congress
                                             97-14866
                                              CIP

97 98 99 00 01 / 9 8 7 6 5 4 3 2 1

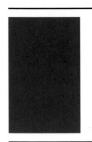

REVIEWERS

SHERRY ARNDT, RN, MPA
Coordinator, Nurse Examiner Program
YWCA
Grand Rapids, Michigan

JAMIE FERRELL, RN, BSN, CEN
Director, Emergency/Trauma Services
Sexual Assault Nurse Examiners Program
Northwest Texas Healthcare System
Amarillo, Texas

JULIE ROSOF, RN, MSN
Family Nurse Practitioner
Assistant in the Department of Community Pediatrics
Vanderbilt University School of Medicine
Nashville, Tennessee

PREFACE

This *Color Atlas of Sexual Assault* provides a critical visual aid in the examination of patients who report having been sexually assaulted. Because the care of this patient requires a multidisciplinary team, the *Atlas* is essential for nurses, nurse examiners, physicians, pathologists, medical examiners, clinical forensic professionals, attorneys, and law enforcement officials.

The photographs were selected from the oral, genital, perianal, and skin variations of thousands of patients of sexual assault. References were chosen from the literature to reflect the current knowledge base. Some of the references are dated, reflecting the need for research into content areas related to sexual assault. The authors are experienced clinicians and have frequently been called as expert witnesses in litigated cases of sexual assault.

The *Atlas* begins with diagrams and photos of the normal genital, perianal, and oral anatomy of adult and adolescent females and males. The physiological changes during the human sexual response are reviewed as are the expected changes that occur in the aging female genitalia.

Chapter 2 presents photographic findings present in sexual assault. These magnified (×15) and 35mm photographs include the external

genitalia, vagina, cervix, external anus and anoscopic views, the oral cavity, and various sites on the skin of the adult, adolescent, and elderly female. Case studies of adult and adolescent females and males show several photographic findings from each of the patients. Findings found after consensual intercourse demonstrate that injury is less prevalent than it is in nonconsensual intercourse, but that consent does not preclude injury.

Chapter 3 consists of photographs of variations of the genitalia, anus and oral cavity caused by infection, surgery, or other variations. These findings may be differentiated from findings consistent with nonconsensual sexual contact, as the reader compares them with photographs in Chapter 2.

Chapter 4 describes the goals of the examiner in providing emotional care, collecting forensic evidence, concluding the acute examination with the patient, and conducting the follow-up examination. Rape trauma syndrome and posttraumatic stress disorder are described. Techniques of critical incident stress debriefing are also described, so that the examiner may integrate these techniques during the medical-legal examination. The medical-legal examination is described according to the California

Office of Criminal Justice Planning (OCJP) Guidelines and based on the adult female model. The California guidelines are currently being revised. The American Society for Testing Materials (ASTM) is preparing guidelines to standardize the examination nationwide. Examination techniques are described for the adolescent and elderly female and also for the adult and adolescent male. Special techniques such as colposcopy are also described. The examiner concludes by teaching, treating by offering medications, connecting the patient to support systems, and checking the evidence collected in the examination. The follow-up examination is emphasized as an essential method to differentiate acute findings from normal variations.

Case Analysis in Chapter 5 provides the reader with an opportunity to make his or her own assessment based on a set of photos. Actual findings are presented for comparison. Case outcome and perpetrator type are identified.

Chapter 6 describes guidelines for the examiner to prepare and provide testimony.

The glossary includes anatomical structures, findings, and related terms. The term *patient* rather than victim or survivor is used to emphasize the objective perspective of the examiner. The term *victim* is used more typically by law enforcement and the judicial system. *Survivor* is used by counselors to indicate that the patient has attained a certain stage of emotional recovery.

The *Atlas* provides an unmatched clinical resource, useful in the medical-legal examination of female and male adult, adolescent, and elderly patients who report being sexually assaulted. However, examination techniques and variations in tissue flexibility and photographic and colposcopic techniques make photographs an approximation of what may be visualized clinically. The *Atlas* photographs are colposcopic magnification at ×15 unless indicated as a 35mm photograph. *Right* and *left* refer to the right and left sides of the patient, not to the sides of the photograph.

ACKNOWLEDGMENTS

Palomar-Pomerado Health System and San Luis Obispo General Hospital supported the Sexual Assault Response Teams that developed this Color Atlas. A special thanks goes to Beverly Miller, RN, Toby Meltzer, MD, and Mary Spencer, MD, for their help and photographs.

Barbara W. Girardin, RN, PhD
Diana K. Faugno, RN, BSN, CPN, BCFE
Patty C. Seneski, RN, ENP
Laura Slaughter, MD, FACR, FACP
Margaret Whelan, RN, BSN

CONTENTS

Detailed Contents

COLOR ATLAS OF SEXUAL ASSAULT

1 ANATOMY AND THE HUMAN SEXUAL RESPONSE

Understanding normal genital, perianal, and oral anatomy, as well as the anatomy and physiology of the human sexual response, provides the basis for evaluating the findings that occur in sexually assaulted patients.

GENITAL ANATOMY

Female Adult and Adolescent

Figure 1-1 is an anatomical diagram of the female genitalia with each anatomical site labeled. The glossary at the end of the text

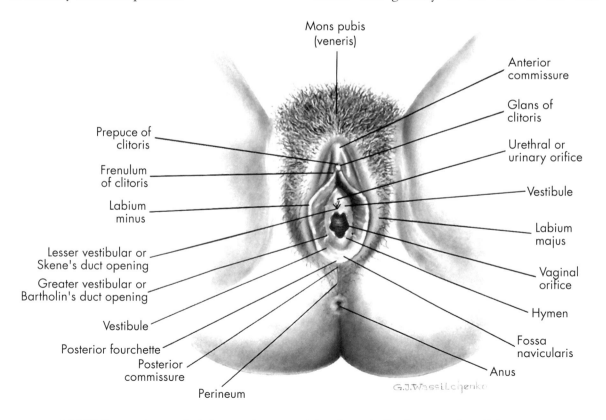

Mons pubis (veneris)

Anterior commissure

Glans of clitoris

Prepuce of clitoris

Urethral or urinary orifice

Frenulum of clitoris

Vestibule

Labium minus

Labium majus

Lesser vestibular or Skene's duct opening

Greater vestibular or Bartholin's duct opening

Vaginal orifice

Hymen

Vestibule

Posterior fourchette

Fossa navicularis

Posterior commissure

Anus

Perineum

G.J.Wassilchenko

FIGURE 1-1 Anatomical sites on the external female genitalia. *(From Lowdermilk DL, Perry SE, Bobak IM:* Maternity and women's health care, *ed 6, St Louis, 1997, Mosby.)*

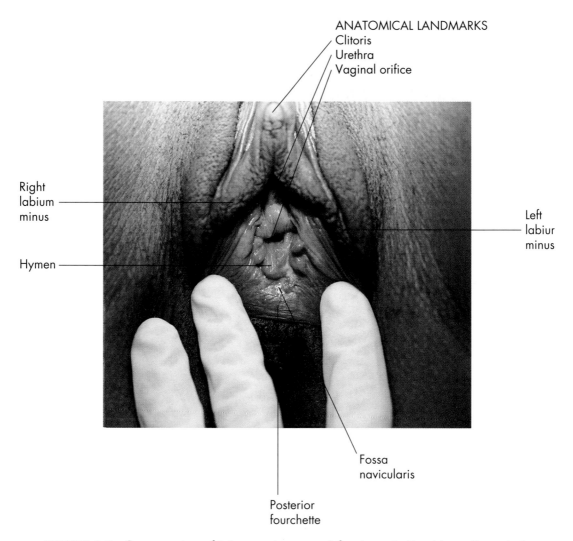

ANATOMICAL LANDMARKS
Clitoris
Urethra
Vaginal orifice

Right labium minus

Left labiur minus

Hymen

Fossa navicularis

Posterior fourchette

FIGURE 1-2   Common sites of injury to the external female genitalia with penile vaginal penetration when the victim is in a supine position (35mm).

describes each of these sites. Identified on Figure 1-2 are the most common sites of injury in nonconsensual penile vaginal penetration when the patient is supine.

The hymen has many normal configurations. The hymen, is a "collar" or "semi-collar" of tissue surrounding the vaginal orifice. It is not a closed door sealing off the vaginal orifice. Most typical configurations are crescentic and annular. Hymens may also be described as redundant and/or fimbriated. The congenital absence of a hymen has never been reported (Jenny, Kunhs, 1987). Hymenal variations include microperforate, imperforate, septate, and cribriform. Age,

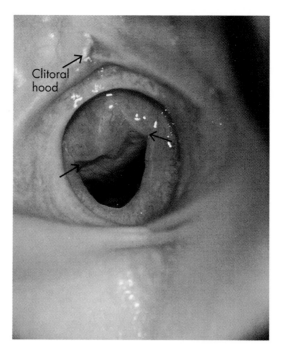

FIGURE 1-3   Crescentic hymen; white, prepubertal (×15).

positioning, degree of relaxation and stage of sexual development affect the appearance of the hymen (Heger, Emans, 1992).

The common crescentic hymen (Figure 1-3) attaches at 1 o'clock or 2 o'clock and extends around 9 o'clock, 10 o'clock, or 11 o'clock, forming a "semi-collar." The hymenal tissue is absent in the suburethral area. The annular hymen in Figure 1-4 is a collar that completely encircles the vaginal orifice, although there may be a normal cleft at 11 o'clock, 12 o'clock, or 1 o'clock.

Before estrogen stimulation, which begins around menarche, the hymen is thin tissue and

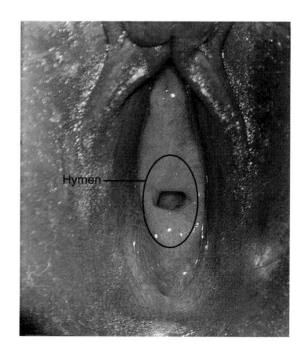

FIGURE 1-4   Annular/circumferential hymen; African-American, prepubertal (×15).

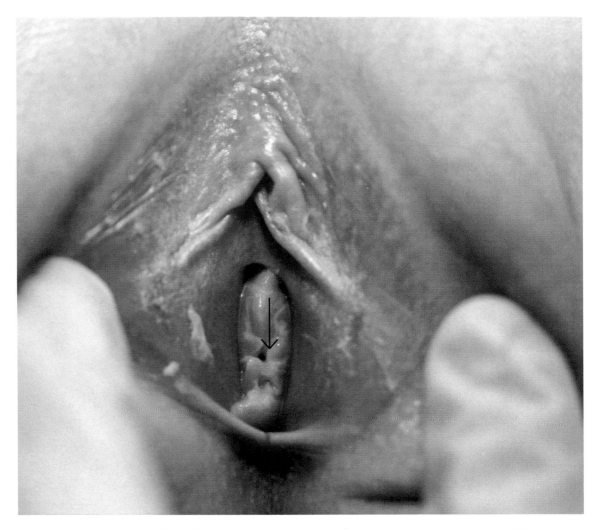

FIGURE 1-5 Fimbriated hymen with white margins from estrogen stimulation; white, Tanner Scale Stage 2, 13-year-old (35mm).

has translucent edges. Mounds or projections on the hymen are common and are associated with vaginal structures such as ridges and posterior columns. The hymen may have tiny scallops, and it is fimbriated (Pokorny, 1992) (Figure 1-5).

With adult estrogen stimulation, the hymen becomes redundant. It is characterized by abundant tissue folded over itself (Figure 1-6). The sleevelike hymen in Figure 1-7 is annular, redundant, and protruding. In sexually active females, hymenal clefts are common but the semblance of a collar remains (Figure 1-8). Perivestibular support bands may be present at the urethra or hymen. They are structures supporting the pelvic floor. Periurethral support bands are present in Figure 1-9. They have a feathering appearance on both sides of the urethra.

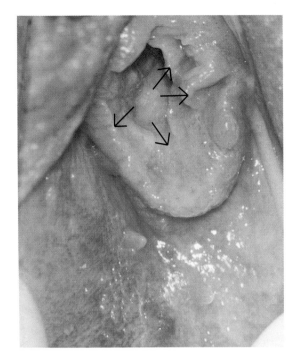

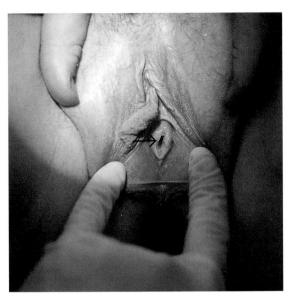

FIGURE 1-6   Redundant hymen; white, sexually inactive 14 year old (×15).

FIGURE 1-7   Sleevelike, redundant, annular hymen; white, sexually inactive 14 year old (35mm).

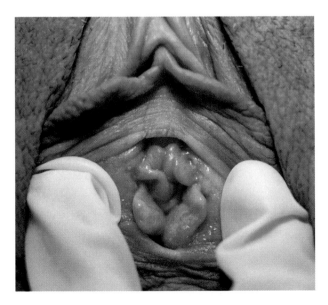

FIGURE 1-8   Redundant hymen; African-American, sexually active 20 year old. The pubic hair is shaved laterally (35mm).

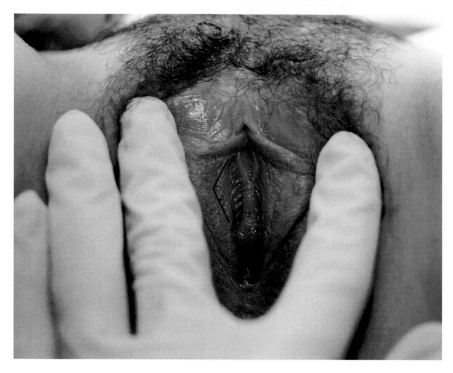

FIGURE 1-9 Periurethral support bands on both sides of the urethra (35mm). Bands are evident on the patient's left side with retraction of the labia.

Puberty begins in females between approximately 8 and 13 years and may take several years to complete. The physical changes of puberty occur in an orderly sequence, but the onset may vary due to general health and nutrition, socioeconomic conditions, and genetic factors (West, 1990). Under the influence of increasing ovarian estrogen, the vaginal epithelium increases in thickness, vaginal secretions acidify, and the labia majora and minora become larger and fuller. The hymen becomes larger, thicker, and redundant, and has blanched edges. Of 200 sexually inactive adolescents, 62% had annular hymens, 38% had crescentic hymens, and 70% had redundant hymens (Emans and others, 1994). A white margin on the fimbriated hymen is a sign of beginning es-

trogen stimulation (Figure 1-5). Vestibular papulations (Figure 1-10) may be present in the adolescent. Papillation can not be differentiated anatomically from genital warts of human papilloma virus (HPV). The vaginal orifice and clitoris enlarges. There is axillary hair growth and a redistribution of adipose tissue. The pubic hair begins to develop during adolescence (Carpentar, Ruck, 1992). The Tanner Scale categorizes female secondary sexual development based on pubic hair pattern and breast development (Tanner, 1962) (see Chapter 4, Table 4-2, pp. 111-113).

The vaginal wall should be pink with rugation (Figure 1-11). The cervix should be pink, smooth and evenly colored (Figure 1-12). The cervical lips consist of stratified squamous ep-

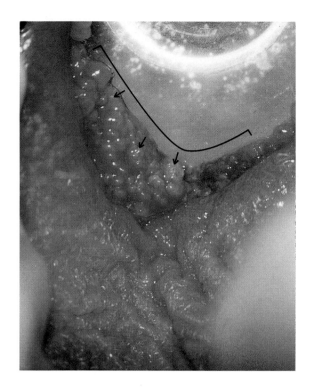

FIGURE 1-10 Vestibular papillae (hymenal) (×15). The inflated balloon present in the introitus is used to examine the contour of the hymen.

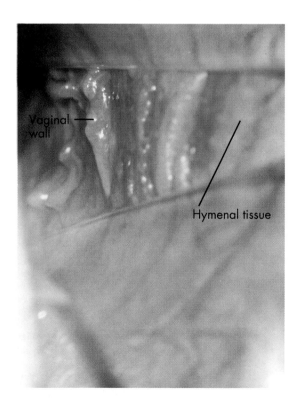

FIGURE 1-11 Normal left vaginal wall, viewed through the side of a clear vaginal speculum (×15).

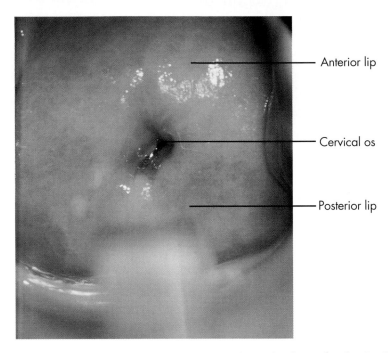

— Anterior lip

— Cervical os

— Posterior lip

FIGURE 1-12   Nulliparous cervix (×15). Opacity along the lower border is the vaginal speculum.

ithelium. The cervical canal, to which the cervical os is the opening, consists of unstratified, columnar epithelium. There may be a circumscribed area around the cervical os of exposed columnar epithelium from the cervical canal. This is called ectropion or eversion (Figure 1-13) and is a common finding in women of all ages (Bowers, Thompson, 1992). Figure 1-14 are some of the common variations in the appearance of the cervix.

Aging Changes in the Elderly Female

The average age of menopause in the United States is 51.4 years (Scott and others, 1994) with a strong genetic factor affecting the age of onset when menstruation ceases. The transitional period during which the reproductive functions decline are caused by diminishing ovarian estrogen levels. The transitional period usually be-

gins 3 to 5 years before menopause. Estrogen is present in menopause but in reduced amounts compared with premenopausal concentrations. Postmenopausal circulating estrogen comes from ovarian and adrenal androgens that are converted to estrogen peripherally (West, 1990). There is enough estrogen to support the health of the genital tissues, although menstrual cycling ceases. Aging changes in the genitalia may be less bothersome if the woman has regular sexual stimulation either through intercourse or manual genital stimulation, or has estrogen therapy (Masters, Johnson, 1966).

Thinning of the hair over the mons pubis and the labia majora occurs, subcutaneous fatty tissues decreases, and the labial folds flatten or disappear (Figure 1-15). The inner surfaces of the labia majora and minor are more pale and dry than in women of childbearing age. The clitoris

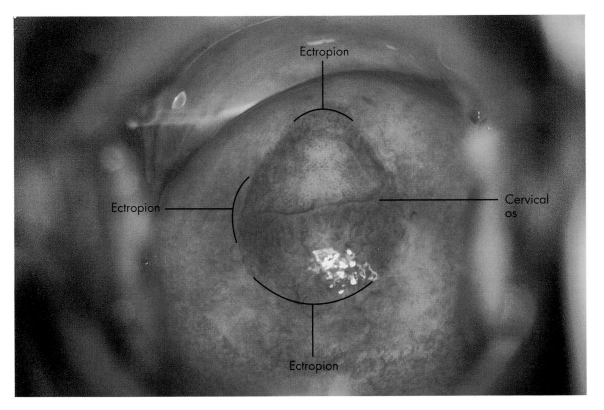

FIGURE 1-13   Ectropion around a parous cervical os (×15).

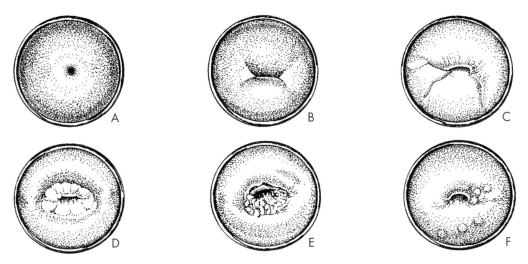

FIGURE 1-14   Common appearances of the cervix. **A,** Nulliparous cervix; **B,** Parous cervix; **C,** Multigravidas, lacerated; **D,** Ectropion or everted; **E,** Eroded; **F,** Nabothian cysts. *(From Seidel HM et al:* Mosby's guide to physical examination, *ed 3, St Louis, 1995, Mosby.)*

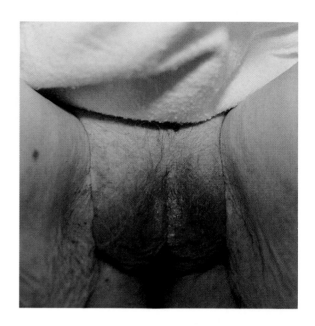

FIGURE 1-15 Flattening of labial folds and thinning of hair; white, 83-year-old (35mm).

is slightly smaller as a result of declining estrogenic stimuli. The urethral meatus may be irregularly located closer to the vaginal introitus as a result of the relaxation of the perineal muscles. The vaginal introitus itself may be smaller in women with declining estrogenic stimuli, admitting only one finger for examination (Barber, 1988). In multiparous women, it may gape open (Figure 1-16) because of relaxation of the muscles of the pelvic floor.

The vagina actually shortens and narrows, and the color is more pale than in the premenopausal female. There is a loss of the superficial layers of the vaginal epithelium. Rugae diminish with age leaving the vaginal walls smooth, thin, shiny, and less elastic. There may be less vaginal mucous than in younger females (Nachtigall, 1994).

The cervix is diminished in size, but should be nontender, and should be evenly rounded and firm, similar to the tip of the nose. There is less protrusion into the vaginal vault, giving the appearance that the cervix is actually flush with the walls. The vaginal fornices also diminish and then disappear because the cervix protrudes less. The cervical os may be narrowed, stenosed, or even obliterated.

The perianal folds may show an increase in pigmentation, with coarse skin. Anal sphincter tone, control and sensation may be diminished. The walls of the anal canal should be smooth and nontender.

The decrease in lubrication, subcutaneous fat, and increased fragility of the tissues in the elderly (Danforth, Scott, 1986) increases the probability of genital injury in sexual assault (Cartwright, 1987). However the type and sites of injury in the elderly in nonconsensual intercourse is typical of that found in nonconsensual intercourse in premenopausal women, as estimated in a group of 30 elderly, sexually assaulted patients (Seneski, 1996).

Male Adult and Adolescent

The two major parts of the male genitalia are the penis and the scrotum. The penis is composed of the penile shaft, which is the cylindric part. The glans is the enlarged region on the

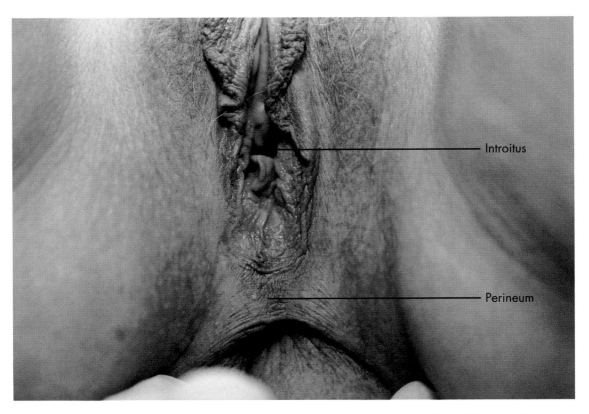

FIGURE 1-16   Gaping, multiparous introitus with a sagging perineum in an Hispanic 68-year-old (35mm).

distal end of the penis, which contains the urethral orifice (Figure 1-17). The foreskin or prepuce is the loosely fitting skin covering the glans. It may be partially or totally removed in the circumcised male. The scrotum is the double sac containing the testes, part of the spermatic cord, and muscles. Semen is composed of spermatozoa from the testes and seminal fluid from the prostate.

Impaired spermatogenesis may occur from environmental toxins, undescended testes, traumatic or infection-related testicular atrophy, alcohol or marijuana use, prolonged fever, and endocrine disorders. Antispermatozoa antibodies may cause oligospermia.

Defective delivery of sperm into the vagina may be caused by obstruction of the seminal tract as a result of inflammation or infection (West, 1990).

Puberty in males begins between 9 and 14 years. The influences of testosterone on the genitalia are growth of the penis and prostatic seminal vesicles, secretory activity of the prostate and seminal vesicles, maturation of germ cells, development of the rugae pattern, and darkening of scrotal skin (West, 1990). The Tanner Scale categorizes secondary sexual development in the male based on pubic hair, penis and scrotum characteristics (Tanner, 1962) (see Chapter 4, Table 4-3, pp. 117-118).

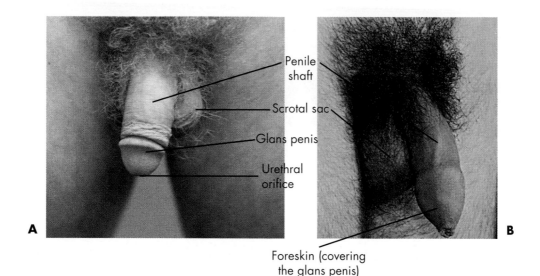

FIGURE 1-17   Male genitalia. **A**, Circumcised; **B**, Uncircumcised. *(From Seidel HM et al: Mosby's guide to physical examination, ed 3, St Louis, 1995, Mosby.)*

THE HUMAN SEXUAL RESPONSE

The human sexual response prepares for non-traumatic intercourse (Masters, Johnson, 1966). Table 1-1 describes the human sexual response in four stages for females and males.

The normal sexual response is typically absent in the victim during the sexual assault. There is no pelvic tilt, partner assistance with insertion, increase in lubrication, or relaxation (Slaughter, 1995), which explains why genital injury may occur in sexual assault. In spousal rape, the normal sexual response may occur to some degree and therefore injury may be limited or absent.

Elderly Female

The elderly female has changes in the normal sexual response to sexual stimulation. The excitement phase is shorter both in time and the extent of the expansion of the vagina than in younger women. Vaginal lubrication in women beyond 60 years of age may take from 1 to 3 minutes as compared with the 10 to 30 seconds in younger women (Masters, Johnson, 1966). However, in women who have continued to have sexual intercourse once or twice a week for their entire mature lives, rapid and full lubrication may occur despite atrophy and thinning of the vaginal walls (Masters, Johnson 1966).

Diminished vasocongestion of the labia minora and reduced uterine elevation characterizes the aging changes of the plateau phase. The orgasmic phase is shorter and the number of uterine contractions diminishes. Dilatation of the cervical os does not occur in the elderly female as a result of orgasm (Bowers, Thompson, 1992). Occasionally, a spasm of the uterine muscles causes pain. The final phase of resolution is more rapid in older women than in younger women.

Table 1-1 *Human sexual response in females and males*

PHASES	FEMALE RESPONSE	MALE RESPONSE
EXCITEMENT Develops from somatic or psychological stimuli	Genital and generalized vasocongestion and myotonia Clitoral tumescence; vaginal lubrication primarily from transudate through the vaginal wall; Bartholin glands and cervical mucous produce only negligible lubrication	General vasocongestion and myotonia Penile tumescence from average flaccid length of 8.5 cm to erect length of 16 to 19 cm; flaccid circumference average 3.0 cm to erect average circumference of 3.5 cm Testes elevate as a result of shortening of the spermatic cords.
PLATEAU Sexual tension intensifies; duration varies with desire and stimulation	Uterus elevates, tilts back and the fundus contracts to form a reservoir for sperm; inner two thirds of vagina distend from 2 cm wide × 7.5 cm long to 5.75 cm wide × 10.5 cm long, ventrally Vagina is distensible to accommodate the delivery of full-term head (32 to 36 cm circumference) Labia minora engorge, adding 1 cm to the length of the vagina, removing the anatomical cover, and providing a penile support	Diameter of glans penis increases to an average of 3.5 cm Neither muscular development nor flaccid size relate to erect penile size. Nether circumcision nor age automatically lead to impotence Scrotum becomes vasocongested; testes continue to engorge and elevate
ORGASMIC Vasocongestion and myotonia are released; lasts a few seconds	Consists of regularly recurring contractions Confined to the outer one third of the vagina and is variable in intensity and duration	Ejaculation of 2 to 7 ml of seminal fluid containing sperm > 20 million/mL. In retrograde ejaculation the fluid may be discharged into the bladder; common after prostatectomy The rectal sphincter contracts sporadically
RESOLUTION Involuntary period of tension loss; returns the person through plateau and excitement to an unstimulated state	Muscle relaxation; cervical os remains dilated 20 to 30 minutes; anterior vaginal wall collapses, placing cervix into sperm pool; can return to another orgasm any time during resolution	Muscle relaxation; refractory period after resolution prohibits return to orgasm

Adapted from Masters WH, Johnson VE: *The human sexual response*, Boston, 1966, Little Brown.

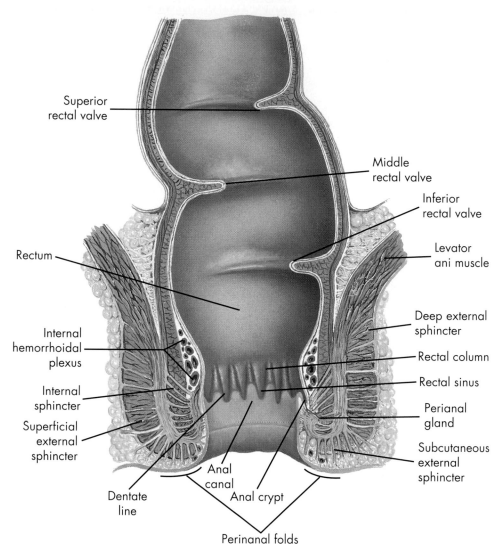

FIGURE 1-18   Anal and rectal anatomy. *(From Seidel HM et al:* Mosby's guide to physical examination, *ed 3, St Louis, 1995, Mosby.)*

PERIANAL ANATOMY

Major perianal anatomical sites are identified in Figure 1-18. Moving from the outside to the inside, there is the perianal area, which is roughly circular and includes the anal folds-furrowed area of skin covering the involuntary muscle of the anus (Figure 1-19). The skin is more pigmented and more coarse than the skin on the buttocks. There is a change in pigment with age and in different ethnic groups. The perianal area is delicate and pain sensitive (West, 1990). Figure 1-20 shows an anal tag at 12 o'clock.

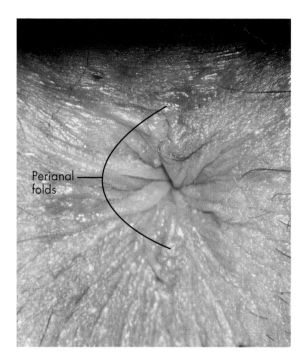

FIGURE 1-19 Normal perianal area and anus (×15).

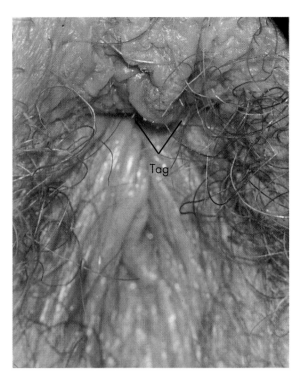

FIGURE 1-20 Anal tag at 12 o'clock on the perianal folds (×15).

The anus is a slit, opening into the anal canal. The anal canal is a distensible passageway of about 3 cm long that links the exterior of the body at the anus to the rectum at the dentate line. The external part of the anal canal is made of delicate sensitive skin. The internal part of the canal is lined with pain-insensitive mucous membrane. The tissue is pink-to-salmon–color and free of lesions, as shown by the anoscopic view in Figure 1-21. Surrounding the anal canal are the internal and external anal sphincters. The dentate line is the superior boundary of the anal canal, where the rectal columns interconnect with anal papilla (Clemente, 1985). Superior to the dentate line is the rectum.

The anal sphincteric ring encircles the anal canal. It is composed of components of the voluntary external sphincter, the levator and longi-

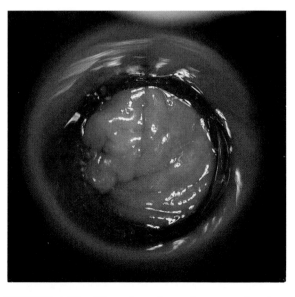

FIGURE 1-21 Normal anal canal, anoscopic view. Anoscope is inserted fully. There is lubricating jelly and some stool present (×15).

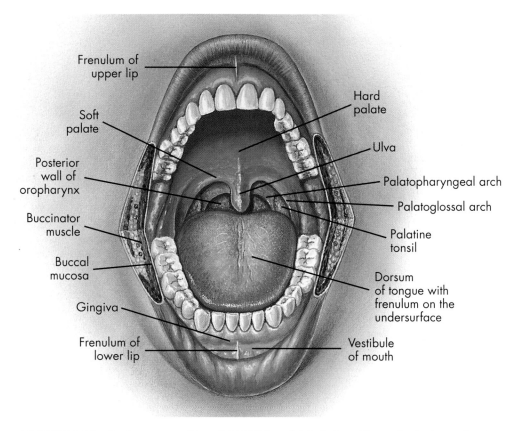

FIGURE 1-22 Oral anatomy. *(From Seidel HM et al: Mosby's guide to physical examination, ed 3, St Louis, 1995, Mosby.)*

tudinal muscles and the involuntary internal sphincter. The external sphincter is a striated muscle that wraps around the internal sphincter. The external sphincter extends the entire length of the anal canal. The external sphincter relaxes from its usual contracted position for defecation. At rest, the sphincter should be contracted and the anus should be closed. During examination, the anal sphincter tightens, resisting the insertion of an examining finger. The anterior portion of the sphincteric ring is more vulnerable to trauma (West, 1990).

The rectum lies superior to the dentate line and lies between the anal canal and the sigmoid flexure of the large intestine. It is about 13 cm long. The lining of the rectum consists of red, glistening, glandular mucosa. The rectal mucosa has autonomic nerve supply and is relatively pain insensitive. Small foreign bodies may lodge at the dentate line. Foreign bodies will reach the rectum if they are fully inserted and are greater than 3 cm long—the length of the anal canal.

ORAL ANATOMY

The examination sites in the oral cavity are identified in Figure 1-22. The lips are consistent in color and may have dry or cracked opposing surfaces. The buccal mucosal, hard and soft palate, and tongue are each uniformly pink and free of lesions. The dorsum of the tongue is covered by papillae, which appear rough. A thin white coating is not uncommon. The undersurface of the tongue is smooth with evident blood vessels and an intact frenulum. Above and behind the tongue are two arches—the palatoglossal and palatopharyngeal—supported by their respective pillars. These vertical portions of the arches are also called the anterior and posterior pillars. The tonsils can be seen in the cavities, between the pillars. At the center of the palatoglossal arch is the uvula. The posterior pharynx may normally have small blood vessels and patches of lymphoid tissue present. In the adult, there are 32 teeth, including the third molars or wisdom teeth (Clemente, 1985).

Sites that are prone to injury in oral copulation are the vermilion and mucosal surface of the lips, frenula, hard and soft palate, palatoglossal arch, and uvula.

REFERENCES

Barber HR: *Geriatric gynecology.* New York, 1988, MacMillan.

Bowers AC, Thompson J: *Clinical manual of health assessment,* ed 4, St Louis, 1992, Mosby.

Cartwright PS: Factors that correlate with injury sustained by survivors of sexual assault, *Ob Gyn* 70:44, 1987.

Carpenter SE, Ruck J, editors: *Pediatric and adolescent gynecology,* New York, 1992, Raven Press.

Clemente CD, editor: *Gray's anatomy,* ed 37, New York, 1985, Churchill-Livingstone.

Danforth DN, Scott JR, editors: *Obstetrics and gynecology,* ed 5, Philadelphia, 1986, JP Lippincott

Emans SJ and others: Hymenal findings in adolescent women: impact of tampon use and consensual sexual activity, *J Pediatr* 125:153, 1994.

Jenny C, Kunhs ML: Hymens in newborn female infants, *Pediatr* 80:399, 1987.

Heger AH, Emans SJ: *Evaluation of the sexually abused child,* New York, 1992, Oxford.

Masters WH, Johnson VE: *The human sexual response,* Boston, 1966, Little Brown.

Nachtigall LE: Sexual function in menopause and postmenopause, In Lobo, RA: *Treatment of postmenopausal women: basic and clinical aspects,* New York, 1994, Raven Press.

Pokorny S: Anatomical terms of female external genitalia. In Heger AH, Emans SJ, editors: *Evaluation of the sexually abused child,* New York, 1992, Oxford.

Seneski PC: Rape in the elderly female. Paper presented at the Sexual Assault Examiner Training Course, Palm Springs, Calif, March, 1996.

Scott JR and others, editors: *Danforth's obstetrics and gynecology,* ed 7, Philadelphia, 1994, JB Lippincott.

Slaughter L: Medical examination: the state protocol. Paper presented at Certification Course for Sexual Assault Response Team (SART), San Diego, January, 1995.

Tanner JM: *Growth at adolescence,* ed 2, Oxford, 1962, Blackwell Scientific.

West JB, editor: *Best and Taylor's Physiological basis of medical practice,* ed 12, Baltimore, 1990, Williams and Wilkins.

SUGGESTED READING

Gebhard PH, Johnson AB: *The Kinsey data: marginal tabulations of the 1938–1963 interviews conducted by the Institute for Sex Research,* Philadelphia, 1979, WB Saunders.

2 FINDINGS IN SEXUAL ASSAULT AND CONSENSUAL INTERCOURSE

DEFINITION AND INCIDENCE OF SEXUAL ASSAULT

Sexual assault involves a wide range of behaviors that involve unwanted sexual contact. The term sexual assault includes sexual contact, as in fondling, and sexual penetration, as in rape. Sexual assault or rape may be classified according to the victim as child sexual assault, incest, marital rape, and male rape. The assault may also be classified according to the perpetrator as date rape, acquaintance rape, and stranger rape. Repeated sexual assault within a relationship is called sexual abuse.

The legal definitions of rape and penetration vary from state to state and is defined by statute. Rape typically involves (1) forced sexual intercourse, (2) psychological coercion, verbal threats, and physical force, and (3) lack of consent (Bureau of Justice Statistics, 1995a). Full erection and ejaculation does not have to occur for rape to have been committed.

Penetration of the vagina, oral cavity, or anus may occur with the penis, fingers, or foreign objects, to both females and males, between marriage partners, persons of the same gender, acquaintances, and strangers (Burgess and others, 1995). Penetration, however slight, of the labia or rectum by the penis, other body part, or foreign object constitutes the act of penetration. The legal definitions of oral copulation and masturbation require only contact with the lips or genitalia respectively (Office of Criminal Justice, 1987).

Rhode Island defines sexual assault by degree:

First degree Sexual penetration by a part of a person's body or by any object into the genital, oral, or anal openings, which occurs when there is: (1) force or coercion, (2) mental or physical inability to communicate and (3) unwillingness to engage in an act.

Second degree Sexual contact without penetration that could include intentional touching of a person's sexual or intimate parts or the victim's clothing covering the intimate parts when there is (1) force or coercion or (2) mental or physical unwillingness to engage in such an act.

Third degree Sexual penetration by a person 18 years or older of a person under the age of consent.

The National Crime Victimization Study (Bureau of Justice Statistics, 1995b) surveyed households and persons over 12 years of age to determine the estimated incidence of sexual assault of any kind including those committed by intimates or family members. These figures

19

Table 2-1 *Incidence of Female and Male Sexual Assault*		
	FEMALES	MALES
Rapes and sexual assaults 1995*	354,670	n/a
Rapes and sexual assaults 1994*	432,700	n/a
Average annual number of reported rapes and sexual assault in 1992-1993	500,200	48,500
Annual rate per 1,000 (age 12 years or greater)	4.6	0.5
Complete rapes	34%	
Attempted rapes	28%	
Sexual assault with injury	9%	
Sexual assault without injury	15%	
Verbal threat rape/sexual assault	13%	
Pregnant prior to sexual assault	2%†	
Sites of penetration		
Vulvar	95%	Anal
Oral	27%	Oral
Anal	6%	Anal and oral
PERPETRATOR		
Lone offender	90%	93%
Acquaintance	53%	54%
Intimate	26%	
Spouse	5%	
Ex-partner or friend	$^5/_{16}$%	
Stranger	18%	46%
Other relative	3%	
Multiple	10%	<10 sample cases
Those surveyed who knew >1 perpetrators	37%	
Those surveyed who knew 0 perpetrators	63%	

From Bureau of Justice Statistics: *National crime victimization survey: preliminary results for 1995*, Washington, DC, 1996, US Department of Justice
*Bureau of Justice Statistics, 1996
†n=5,734; Satin and others, 1991

may be more accurate than the figures based on police reports, which are estimated at 32% of the actual occurrence of female sexual assault (Bureau of Justice Statistics, 1996). Males report sexual assault even less than do females, primarily because of their humiliation in failing to protect themselves (Hickson and others, 1994). Table 2-1 describes some of the findings from the National Crime Victimization Study.

Although sexual assault occurs in all age, race, ethnic, and cultural groups, rape is highest among 20 to 24-year-old black females (Bureau of Justice Statistics, 1995b). Females ages 16 to 19 are the next group most at risk. Other associated factors are prior history of rape or incest, drug and alcohol use, visitor status, homelessness, and mental disability (McCall, 1993). In testing a path, model ($n = 622$), Draucker (1997) showed that negative family health, sexual abuse, and physical maltreatment related to adult victimization. Although certain behaviors may increase a person's risk of victimization, it is the offender who is responsible for the act (Burgess and others, 1995).

Repeated sexual victimization occurred in 66% of 433 sexually assaulted survey respondents ($n = 3,131$) (Sorenson and others, 1991). The average number of victimizations was 3.2. Draucker (1997) demonstrated that initial victimization relates to subsequent victimization in a study of 622 community-based women.

In a study of 2,091 adolescent girls (Hibbard, Ingersoll, Orr, 1990), 12.9% of the girls reported being sexually assaulted. In another study of adolescent girls (Nagy, Adcock, Nagy, 1994), 13% of 1,690 girls reported being sexually assaulted.

Ten percent to 14% of all women have been raped by a spouse (Allison, Wrightsman, 1993). Of women who are physically assaulted by their husbands, 33% to 46% are assaulted sexually (Frieze, Brown, 1989).

Of all those sexually assaulted in 1995, 32% reported the incident (Bureau, 1996). Guilt, fear of retribution, humiliation, lack of knowledge and trust in the legal and medical system and impaired cognitive processing that occurs following the intense trauma of the assault are reasons why those persons assaulted sexually choose not to report (Burgess, Fehder, Hartman, 1995). Coercive sexual intercourse in marriage and in homosexual relationships may be reported less because the assault occurs in domestic circumstances and the perpetrator and victim may have had sexual relations in the past (Hickson and others, 1994)

Perpetrators who are acquaintances are reported more often than perpetrators who are intimates and strangers. In one group of college males, 15% said they had committed acquain-

tance rape, and 11% said they used physical restraints to force a woman to have sex (Rapaport, Posey, 1991). Among this group of college males, 35% admitted that under certain circumstances they would commit rape if they believed they could get away with it. Of college males who committed rape, 84% did not classify it as rape (Koss, Dinero, Seibel, 1988).

Patients having experienced date rape are typically 16 to 19 years old and believe that consensual sex play provoked the nonconsensual intercourse and therefore feel *they* are at fault, not the perpetrator who ignored pleas to stop (Davis, Peck, Storment, 1993). In a survey of 6,159 college students enrolled at 32 institutions in the United States, 54% of women had been the victim of some form of sexual abuse. Of these incidences 57% occurred on dates, while 73% of the perpetrators and 55% of the victims had used alcohol or other drugs prior to the assault (Koss, 1988). In a study of 11 to 14 year olds (White, Humphrey, 1991), 51% of the boys and 41% of the girls said forced sex was acceptable if the boy, "spent a lot of money" on the girl. Sixty-five percent of the boys and 47% of the girls said it was acceptable for a boy to rape a girl if they had been dating for more than 6 months. In the high school group, more boys (76%) than girls (56%) believed forced sex was acceptable under certain circumstances, as when a man and woman were married (White, Humphrey, 1991).

The national incidence of rape in *elderly* females 65 years of age and older was 10 per 100,000 in 1990 (Federal Bureau of Investigation [FBI], 1993). During 1992 this category had increased by 2% (FBI, 1993). Of those over age 50, 60,000 are victimized by rape and sexual assault per year (Ramin and others, 1992).

In a study ($n = 760$) at one inner-city hospital 2.7% of the sexually assaulted patients were 60

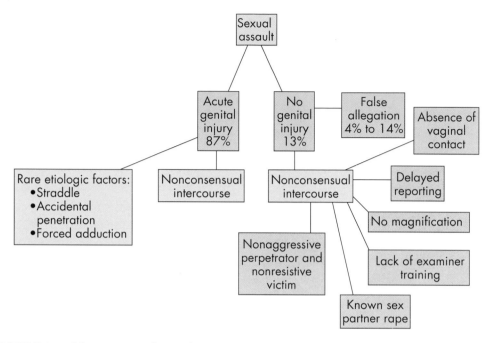

FIGURE 2-1 The presence of genital injury in sexual assault (×15). (NOTE: There are variations in this schema, such as false allegation when injury is present.)

years or older (Cartwright, Moore, 1989). In another study, 2.2% of reported sexual assault cases involved females 50 years or older (Ramin and others, 1992). Many elderly victims lived alone and were assaulted in their homes in the evening by strangers with guns or sharp objects (Bureau of Justice Statistics, 1994). In elderly rapes that occurred in the home, 43% admitted the rapist into their home and 36% of the perpetrators gained access through an open window or door (Tyra, 1993). The motive for rape in the elderly may be revenge against an authority figure (Groth, 1979; Tyra, 1993), or the rape may occur secondary to robbery (Douglas and

others, 1992), with the elderly serving as an accessible, vulnerable target.

FINDINGS IN THE ASSAULTED FEMALE: ADULT AND ADOLESCENT

Figure 2-1 shows that genital injury may or may not be present in sexually assaulted patients, even when examined within 48 hours. The following discussion elaborates on Figure 2-1.

Slaughter and Brown (1992) found genital injury in 87% of the patients reporting within 48 hours after nonconsensual penile vaginal penetration (*n* = 238) when examined by a prepared sexual assault examiner and with colposcopic magnification. Genital injury may be present even when there are no subjective symptoms reported by the patient (Rambow and others, 1992).

Injury occurs in sexually assaulted patients because of multiple factors in the victim and in the perpetrator. The posterior fourchette, labia minora, hymen, and fossa navicularis are the most common sites of injury in penile vaginal penetration (Slaughter, 1997). Injury at these sites suggests that the lack of the human physiological response to sexual stimulation plays a significant role.

In the victim, there is a lack of pelvic tilt and partner assistance with insertion, lack of lubrication, and relaxation (Slaughter, 1995). Lack of pelvic tilt and partner assistance with insertion combined with forced intromission results in injury, especially at the posterior fourchette, labia minora, hymen, and fossa navicularis. Lack of increased lubrication causes abrasion or lacerations with the friction of the opposing forces at the labia minora and hymen, since these parts are pulled inward with the penetrating object. Vaginal lacerations and ecchymosis result from the lack of lubrication of the penetrating force. However lubrication alone, such as menstrual blood, does not protect the external nor internal genitalia from injury during nonconsensual contact (Slaughter, 1995). Lack of cooperation and relaxation creates a less flexible surface against which the offending object forces itself, causing more blunt force trauma such as ecchymosis and swelling.

In the perpetrator, there is generally increased force consistent with this crime of violence. The increased force results in an increased probability of injury. However, the prevalence of serious injury requiring medical care, hospitalization, or surgery is less than 5%, and death in connection with sexual assault is less than 1%. Sexual dysfunction, including impotence, delayed ejaculation, and premature ejaculation (Groth, Burgess, 1977), may prolong the duration of tissue friction and blunt trauma and therefore increase the probability of injury. Excessive force is particularly characteristic of the perpetrator who has a history of, or preference for, anal intercourse and also when the sequence of acts is anal penetration followed by oral penetration (Slaughter, 1996). Attacks outdoors may be more violent than those that occur inside. The relationship between the perpetrator and the victim may also influence the pattern and severity of injury such that the intimate or exintimate present with less injury (Slaughter, 1997).

Physical injury, including genital injury, is not an inevitable consequence of rape and the absence of genital injury does not provide proof of consent (Cartwright, 1987, Douglas and others, 1992; Heger, Emans, 1992; Lauber, Souma, 1982; Slaughter, Brown, 1992). Slaughter and Brown (1992) found 13% of sexually assaulted patients had no genital injury (see Figure 2-1). The absence of genital injury, in the sexually assaulted patient may be explained by several possibilities: the lack of vaginal contact by the perpetrator, delayed reporting, the lack of magnification, the lack of training or experience by the examiner, known sex partner rape, and a nonaggressive perpetrator with a nonresistive victim. False allegation may also be a consideration.

There are reasons for no injury. For example, if the perpetrator had no contact with the vagina, then it follows that there would be no genital injury.

An examination delayed to 14 days postassault will detect no acute findings. In one study of 311 postassault patients, no scars were noted at the 2-week follow-up examination. Figure 2-2 shows the subtle evidence present at 10 days postassault. Even at 72 hours postassault, only 52% of those assaulted will have findings (Slaughter, 1997).

Lack of magnification can drop the probability of detecting injury from 87% with colposcopy and a trained examiner, to 10% to 30% by gross visualization alone. (Slaughter, Brown, 1992). The lack of examiner preparation in the characteristic sites and features of sexual assault injury may result in the failure to detect injury. Few health care providers, including physicians have had training in a medical school, or residency on the subject of sexual abuse (Heger, Emans, 1992). Using an examiner with special preparation, along with colposcopic magnification, is becoming the standard of practice (see Appendix G, *Resources for the Examiner*).

Patients who have experienced known sex partner rape may have no evidence of injury because of kinesthetic memory, lubrication, and other elements of the human sexual response that may be present.

When the perpetrator uses minimal force and the victim is nonresistive, physical injury may be limited or absent. The power rapist usually uses only whatever force he believes is necessary to get his victim to cooperate. This may be only verbal threat or intimidation, especially when the victim does not resist. The victim may be physically unharmed. However, resistance by the victim activates the perpetrator's anger and increased aggression (Groth, 1979).

False allegation of sexual assault may be motivated by the need to conceal consensual intercourse, the need for nurturance, the need for antibiotics to avert possible sexually transmitted diseases (STDs), and in hopes to be tested for acquired immunodeficiency syndrome (AIDS) fol-

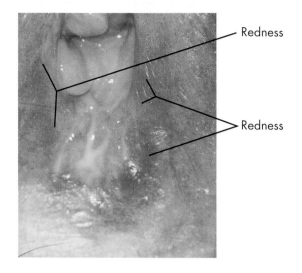

FIGURE 2-2 Delayed examination (×15). This white 22 year old was examined at 10 days postnonconsensual penile vaginal intercourse. Note the residual redness.

lowing unknown exposure. Anger toward the accused perpetrator is another motivation for false allegation, as is the desire to be rescued from ongoing abuse (Aiken, 1993; Feldman, Ford, Stone, 1994; Seneski, 1996). In 1992 the FBI (1993) found that 8% of forcible rapes were unfounded. False allegations have been estimated at 4% in one data base of 2,500 patients examined for sexual assault (Battiste-Otto, 1996) to 10% to 14% (Seneski, 1996) in another data base of 900 patients. Patients with a false allegation of sexual assault typically report within 24 hours of the reported incident (Seneski, 1996; Slaughter, 1997). False allegation may be considered when the findings are inconsistent with the history and time frame, there are no physical or genital injuries and laboratory findings are nonsignificant, or when the patient recants. Recants may result from fear even when assault has occurred.

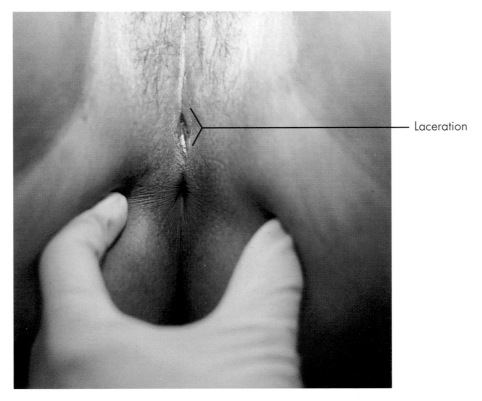

Laceration

FIGURE 2-3 Injury evident on gross visualization (35mm). This white 13 year old presented with a laceration of the posterior fourchette. Laceration extends inward to the fossa navicularis and is evident with separation.

Regardless of whether visible injury is evident, examiners must proceed with the most thorough, nonjudgmental history, physical examination, and evidence collection as is possible. A nonjudgmental attitude helps provide compassionate care and improves the examiners credibility as a witness. The judicial system decides if sexual assault actually occurred based on a multidisciplinary effort of which the examiner's history and examination are a part.

External Genitalia

Much of the injury in sexual assault is difficult to visualize. Although it is small, it is significant. When there is gross injury (Figure 2-3) evident without magnification, it is particularly significant. Of the genital injuries that do occur from forced penile vaginal penetration, 94% have injury to one or more of the first four sites listed in Table 2-2.

The typical types of acute injury to these sites are related to blunt force trauma and can be represented by the acronym TEARS (Slaughter, Brown, 1991):

T Tear (laceration) or tenderness
E Ecchymosis (bruise)
A Abrasion
R Redness (erythema)
S Swelling (edema)

TEARS will be used to represent these five types of injury, which are typical findings in sexual assault. The term "laceration" will be

Table 2-2 *Sites and Type of Genital Injury in Penile Vaginal Penetration*		
SITE	INCIDENCE OF INJURY (%)	TYPES OF INJURY
Posterior fourchette	70	Laceration, abrasion
Labia minora	53	Abrasion, ecchymosis
Hymen	29	Ecchymosis, laceration
Fossa navicularis	25	Laceration, abrasion
Cervix	13	Ecchymosis
Vagina	11	Laceration, ecchymosis
Perineum	11	Laceration, abrasion
Periurethral	9	Ecchymosis
Labia majora	7	Redness, abrasion

From Slaughter L, Brown CRV: Cervical findings in rape victims, *Am J Ob Gyn* 164:528, 1991; Slaughter L: *Personal communication*, December, 1996.

used in place of the "T" in TEARS.

The location of the most common injuries when the perpetrator is superior, occurs where the penis first contacts the perineum. This "mounting injury" is typically on the posterior fourchette from 5 to 7 o'clock and may include lacerations, ecchymosis, abrasion, redness and/or swelling. Figures 2-4 to 2-6 show posterior fourchette injuries. Some lacerations form an arrow (Figure 2-7). No data supports that the direction of force may be concluded from the apex of the arrow (Heger, 1996). Abrasions and ecchymosis are common on the labia minora. Figures 2-8 to 2-12 show labia minora injuries. Hymenal ecchymosis and swelling may be present (Figure 2-13). Swelling is most clear when follow-up photos are compared with those from the acute examination. The hymenal hematoma present in Figure 2-14 appears as ecchymosis in the photograph, but the hematoma was evident by palpation during the examination. Hymenal lacerations (Figure 2-14) are secondary to penetration because the hymen is an internal structure (Gibbons, Vincent, 1992). Hymenal lacerations are not explained by nonpenetrating causes.

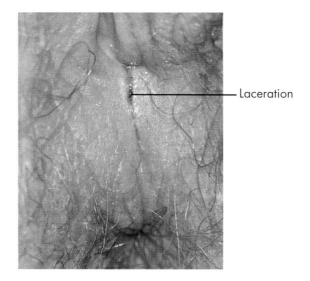
— Laceration

FIGURE 2-4 Posterior fourchette laceration (×15). (Figures 2-4 to 2-6 are the same patient.) This white 24 year old experienced penile vaginal penetration by a neighbor while restrained supine. Examination was 4 hours postassault.

Adolescents

In one study (Slaughter, Brown, 1991), the frequency of hymenal lacerations was 4% in adults and 25% in adolescents. It was concluded that adolescents and adults are not differentiated by the prevalence of injury sites, the

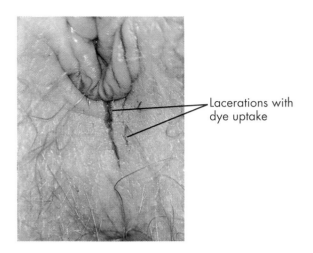

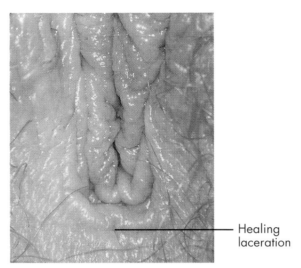

FIGURE 2-5 Posterior fourchette laceration with Toluidine Blue dye uptake (×15). Dye uptake is limited by serous oozing.

FIGURE 2-6 A healing posterior fourchette laceration (×15). No residual TEARS are evident in this examination at 18 days postassault. There was consensual intercourse in a supine position, 30 hours before this examination. There was no evidence of new injury related to the consensual event. OUTCOME: Military court-martial sentenced the perpetrator to 8 to 10 years in prison.

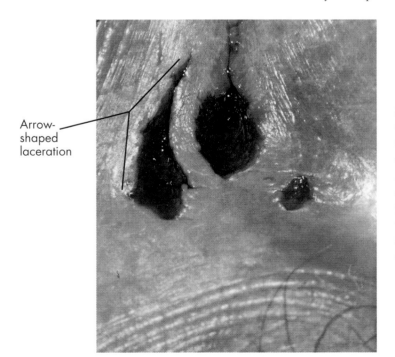

FIGURE 2-7 Posterior fourchette lacerations stained with Toluidine Blue dye (×15). One laceration is in the shape of an arrow. Less dye uptake on the left margin of the middle laceration is a result of oozing. The patient is a white 25 year old who had nonconsensual penile vaginal penetration while restrained supine. OUTCOME: Perpetrator left the country.

Lacerations

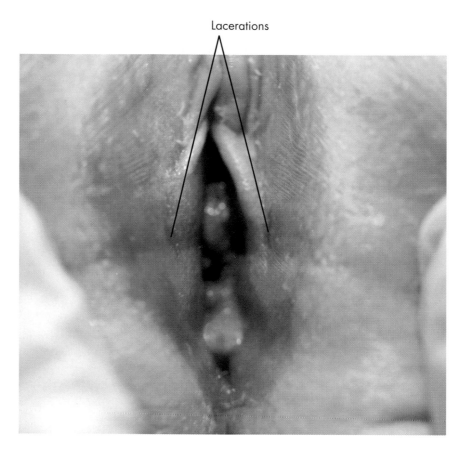

FIGURE 2-8 Labia minora tear (×15). Bilateral linear lacerations on lateral margin of the labia minora from nonconsensual penile vaginal penetration in a supine position. Redness on the right at 7 o'clock to 9 o'clock. Lacerations result from the force of the unlubricated, penetrating object pushing the labial tissue inward. The patient is a white 15 year old.

proportion of single-to-multiple injuries, or in the sites of injury. The only difference in adults and adolescent genital injury is the prevalence of hymenal lacerations which may be explained by the adolescent's sexual inexperience and lack of parity. The hymenal lacerations were single at 6 o'clock or multiple and paired around 6 o'clock. At follow-up the hymenal lacerations did not reunite, and no scarring was evident (Slaughter, 1996).

Elderly

Genital trauma, evident even without colposcopy is more evident in postmenopausal, sexually assaulted patients (age 65 and older), than it is with their younger counterparts (Cartwright, 1987). This may be secondary to the changes that occur with age and the lack of estrogen. However as with those 65 and younger, rape may occur without obvious injury (Cartwright, Moore, 1989; Tyra, 1993). This

Text continues on p. 33.

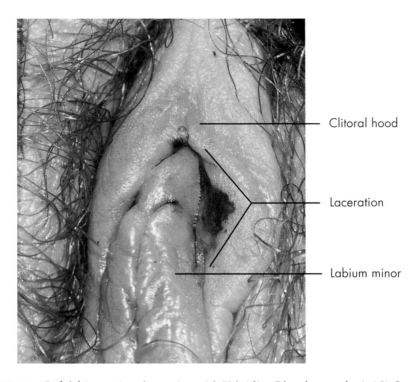

Clitoral hood

Laceration

Labium minor

FIGURE 2-9   Left labium minor laceration with Toluidine Blue dye uptake (×15). Laceration is from 12 to 3 o'clock. Dye uptake is present at the border between the clitoral hood and the labium minor. Redness is from 9 o'clock to 12 o'clock. Swelling is present on the labia minora and right clitoral hood. Swelling and redness are best demonstrated when compared with a similar photo taken at follow-up.

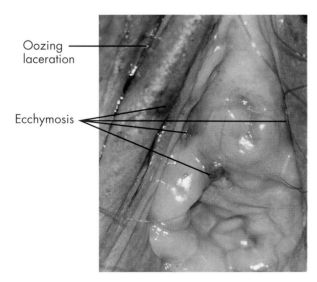

Oozing laceration

Ecchymosis

FIGURE 2-10   Periurethral ecchymosis and swelling (×15). (Figures 2-10 to 2-12 are the same patient.) Ecchymosis is on the periurethral area, hymen, and right labium minor. There is periurethral swelling. Blood is oozing from the labium major laceration. This Asian 23 year old was assaulted in her home by a masked stranger. There was penile and digital vaginal penetration. She was examined 3 hours postassault. OUTCOME: Perpetrator is at large.

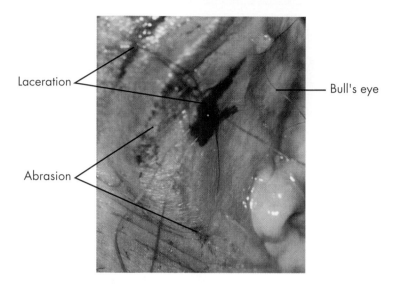

FIGURE 2-11 Circular "bull's eye" ecchymosis of the right labium minus (×15). Bull's eye is from blunt digital force. The blanched center is where the tip of the finger contacts the tissue. The surrounding ecchymosis results from the blood exploding into the tissue around the site of contact. Bleeding lacerations are on the right labium minus and labium major.

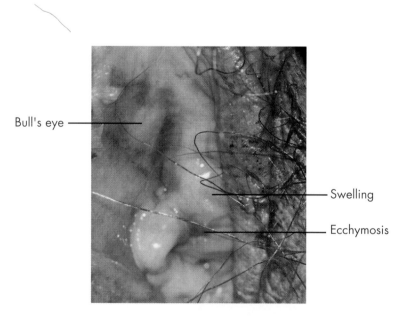

FIGURE 2-12 Circular "bull's eye" close up (×15). Hymenal swelling and ecchymosis is present.

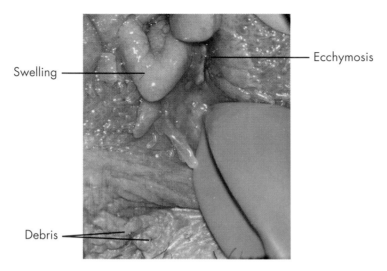

Swelling

Ecchymosis

Debris

FIGURE 2-13 Hymenal swelling and ecchymosis (×15). Hymenal ecchymosis is at 3 o'clock to 5 o'clock. Debris is present on perineum. The green balloon on a cotton-tipped applicator helps provide color contrast. The patient is a white 42 year old who states she is a lesbian. She was assaulted and robbed by two Hispanic males who threatened her with a knife while she was walking her dog in a canyon. OUTCOME: Perpetrators are at large.

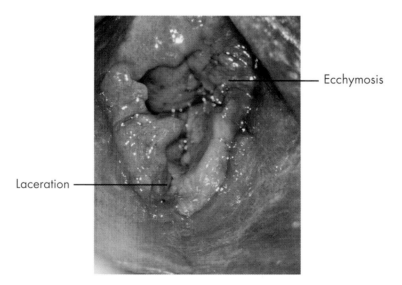

Ecchymosis

Laceration

FIGURE 2-14 Hymenal hematoma (×15). Hematoma is at 1 o'clock to 3 o'clock confirmed by palpation. Hymenal laceration is at 6 o'clock and 7 o'clock within an old transection. There is periurethral swelling. The patient is a Hispanic, 25-year-old, sexually active female. No Toluidine Blue dye has been applied.

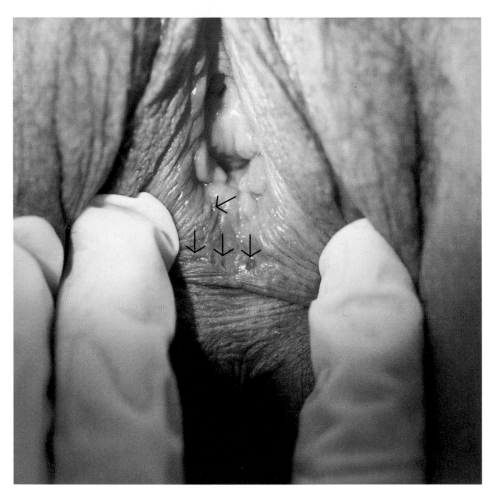

FIGURE 2-15 Fossa navicularis and posterior fourchette lacerations (35mm). (Figures 2-15 and 2-16 are the same patient). Fossa redness and several lacerations from penile vaginal penetration in this white, parous 58 year old. OUTCOME: Perpetrator is at large.

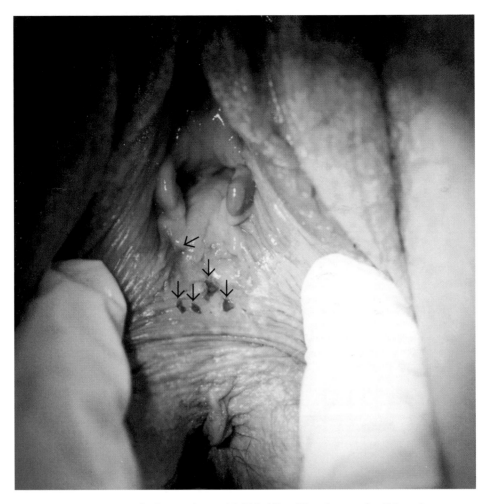

FIGURE 2-16 Lacerations with Toluidine Blue dye uptake (35mm).

was evidenced by the presence of sperm in six sexually inactive elderly patients reporting sexual assault but having no physical or genital injury (Cartwright, Moore, 1989).

In the elderly, penetration of the vagina occurs more often than penetration of the anus. Abrasions and edema were twice as frequent and lacerations were four times more frequent in the elderly group (Cartwright, Moore, 1989). The abrasions along the vaginal walls in postmenopausal assaulted patients may result from

vaginal atrophy (Norvell, Benrubi, Thompson, 1984). Sperm were found in 28% of those elderly examined. Motile sperm were detected only if examined within 6 hours of the assault, compared with detecting motile sperm at 24 hours in the younger group (Ramin and others, 1992).

Figures 2-15 and 2-16 show lacerations of the fossa navicularis and posterior fourchette. Note on the second photograph, that the hymen is flattened posteriorly from greater tension during separation.

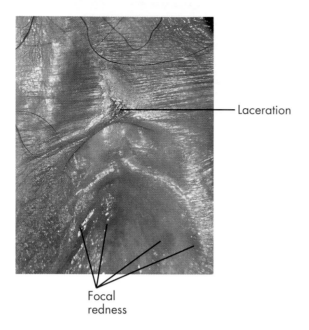

Laceration

Focal
redness

FIGURE 2-17 Clitoral hood laceration and focal redness (×15). Focal redness is inferior to clitoral hood, post digital penetration, on this Hispanic, 20-year-old.

Clitoral injuries are not common from penile penetration. Figures 2-17 to 2-19 show clitoral hood injury secondary to digital contact and suction. Although identifying swelling typically requires a follow up for comparison, the swelling of the clitoral hood in Figure 2-19 is clear when compared with the other side of the clitoral hood.

Infection may also be transmitted during nonconsensual contact, but the risk is small (Jenny and others, 1990). Slaughter and Crowley (1993). found the prevalence of STDs in 170 sex offenders or suspects to be about 7%, which is similar to the rate found in sexually assaulted patients. Trichomoniasis, chlamydia, gonorrhea, and bacterial vaginosis are the infections most commonly diagnosed in patient examinations, but their presence does not represent transmission from the assault if the culture is obtained within 72 hours of the assault (Centers

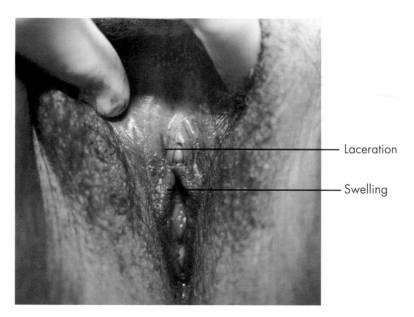

Laceration

Swelling

FIGURE 2-18 Clitoral hood laceration (35mm). Laceration is at the right lateral base of the clitoral hood. There is swelling and redness of the base of the clitoral hood and the superior ends of the labia minora.

for Disease Control and Prevention [CDC], 1993). Evident infection or positive cultures at the time of the examination indicate that the infection antedated the assault. (See Chapter 3 for a description of the major sexually transmitted diseases.)

Vaginal and Cervical Findings

Trauma to the vagina and cervix account for nearly one fourth of all the genital injuries in penile vaginal penetration. (Table 2-2). Cervical injuries, which account for 13% of the injuries, have been reported recently. The increased prevalence of vaginal and cervical injuries may be due in part to the use of magnification. Vaginal lacerations are associated with bleeding, rarely require surgery, and occur in 1% of patients (Geist, 1988). Vaginal lacerations may be more common in older, sexually active, and postmenopausal patients. The examiner should

carefully document the source of the bleeding. Some patients may believe that the bleeding is menstrual bleeding. Figure 2-20 is a vaginal laceration from penetration with a foreign object. Figure 2-21 is injury to the left vaginal wall.

Cervical injury is present in Figures 2-22 to 2-24. The coagulated epithelium present in Figure 2-24 occurs because the epithelial layer at the site of a laceration is detached and dying.

Nonconsensual intercourse may have occurred even without the evidence of semen, which consists of seminal fluid and spermatozoa (Groth, Burgess, 1977). Semen may not be found because of perpetrator and victim factors.

Some perpetrators ejaculate outside of the patient, and some use condoms (Brauner, Gallili, 1993). If ejaculation occurred in the mouth, salivary enzymes rapidly destroy the seminal fluid and its identification after a few hours is difficult (Graves, Sensabaugh, Blake, 1985).

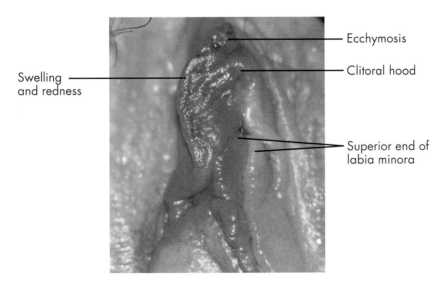

Swelling and redness

Ecchymosis

Clitoral hood

Superior end of labia minora

FIGURE 2-19 Clitoral hood swelling and redness at 9 o'clock to 12 o'clock (×15). Ecchymosis is at 11 o'clock to 12 o'clock. Swelling of the labia minora is present. Injuries are secondary to suction.

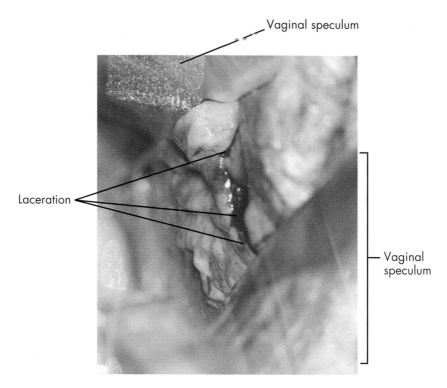

FIGURE 2-20 Left vaginal wall laceration with oozing blood (×15). This white 22 year old was assaulted vaginally with an unidentified foreign object while restrained in a supine position by an unknown male. There was no surgical repair. OUTCOME: Perpetrator is at large.

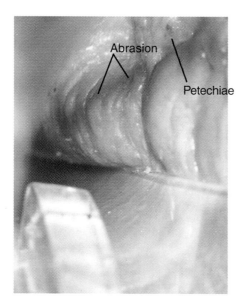

FIGURE 2-21 Left vaginal wall swelling and abrasion (×15). Petechiae are also present. Injury related to penile vaginal penetration.

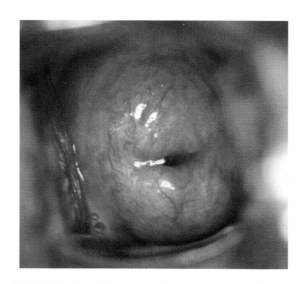

FIGURE 2-22 Hypervascular cervix associated with penile penetration in a Hispanic, sexually active 20 year old (×15). On follow-up at 2 weeks postassault, the hypervascularity had resolved.

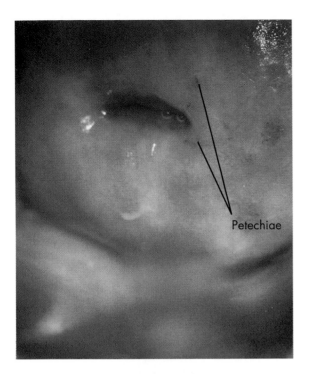

FIGURE 2-23 Cervical redness (×15). Focal areas of redness are at 3 o'clock to 5 o'clock. Petechiae are at 1 o'clock and 4 o'clock near the cervical os. The injury was associated with digital penetration. There was a normal appearance of the cervix at follow-up.

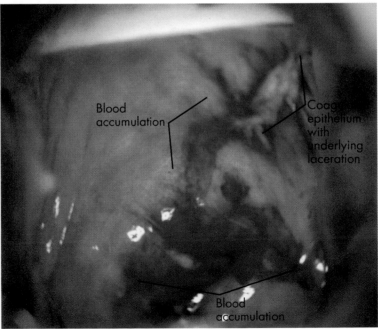

FIGURE 2-24 Cervical laceration (×15). Beneath the coagulated epithelium at 1 o'clock, there is blood oozing from a laceration. The blood is oozing to and around the cervical os, obscuring other lacerations. This 22 year old was examined 6 hours postassault and 4 weeks postuncomplicated vaginal delivery.

Semen may not be found because some perpetrators have retrograde, retarded, or no ejaculation (Douglas and others, 1992; Wissow, 1992). In a study of 170 convicted rapists, Groth and Burgess (1977) reported sexual dysfunction in one third. This is a much higher proportion than is present in the general population. The dysfunction is specific to the assaultive incident, since most reported no sexual dysfunction during consenting intercourse. The most typical sexual dysfunctions were impotence (16%) and retarded ejaculation (15%). Premature ejaculation occurred in 3%. Semen may be lost from the thrusting in and out of the penis after ejaculation or even if the penis remains in the vagina, semen may drain out around the penis.

For the same reasons that semen may not be found, spermatozoa (Figure 2-25) are found in less than half of the patients examined (Ramin and others, 1992). In addition, spermatozoa may not be found if the male is vasectomized, if sperm counts are decreased from alcohol and marijuana use, and if there is delayed reporting. Motile sperm can be detected up to 8 hours postassault from vaginal secretions and up to 72 hours in the endocervical swabs (Secofsky, 1996). Nonmotile spermatozoa persist in the vagina and rectum for up to 24 hours and in the cervical mucus for up to 17 days (Graves, Sensabaugh, Blake, 1985). However sperm quickly lose their tails and they may be difficult to differentiate from debris and yeast cells (Rupp, 1969).

Victim factors contributing to the loss of semen include the lack of sexual response. Without a sexual response the vaginal changes do not occur that should result in the formation of a sperm pool. Obstetrical trauma may also be associated with the loss of semen. Semen may

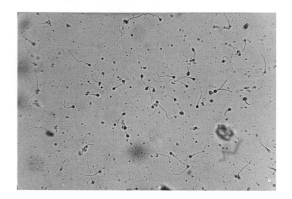

FIGURE 2-25 Sperm, with and without tails, viewed from a light-staining microscope (×74).

have drained out when the patient changed position or walked, or it may have been absorbed by clothing. It then may be detected on skin surfaces or on clothing for hours postassault, if not removed by hygienic activities. Hygienic measures that may result in the loss of semen include wiping, washing, and douching. The patient must be asked these questions because such specifics are not typically volunteered by the patient.

Oral Findings

Forced oral copulation may occur in sexual assault to stimulate an erection in a sexually dysfunctional perpetrator in preparation for vaginal penetration (Groth, Burgess, 1977). The findings in forced oral copulation may be caused from direct trauma, as well as negative pressure (Belizzi, 1980). TEARS may be found on the mucosal, opposing, and vermilion surfaces of the lips and the gums (Figures 2-26 and 2-27). There may be ecchymosis, redness and hypervascularity on the soft and hard palate (Figure 2-28), arches, and uvula (Figure 2-29). Lacerations to either frenulum may indicate

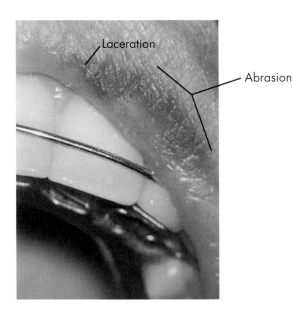

FIGURE 2-26 Upper lip laceration, abrasion, and redness, along the opposing surface of the upper left lip (×15). Laceration is at superior end of abrasion. Patient was a white 26 year old, assaulted in her bedroom at 4 AM. The unidentified male tied her hands with a telephone cord and forced oral copulation. Her retainer was in place at the time of the assault.

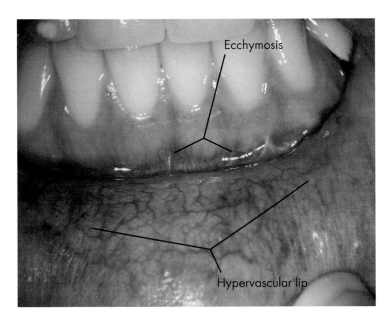

FIGURE 2-27 Ecchymosis of the gums from the frenulum extending left (×10). There is hypervascularity of the lower lip that was absent on follow-up. The frenulum is red and intact. The patient is a white 26 year old who had nonconsensual oral copulation while sitting. The perpetrator was a masked stranger who pushed into her house and threatened her with his knife. He asked her to disrobe, but there was no vaginal nor anal penetration. OUTCOME: Suspect was a serial rapist who is in jail, pending trial.

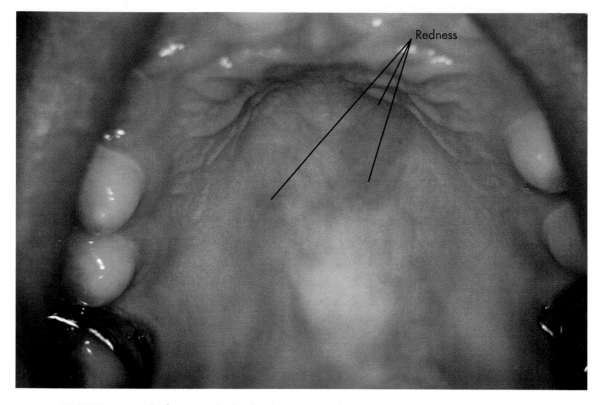

FIGURE 2-28 Redness on the hard palate (×10). This is a white 25 year old. An acquaintance forced oral copulation.

that a foreign object has been forcefully inserted into the mouth.

In the vast majority of consensual oral copulation, there are no lacerations. However, erythema, ecchymosis, swelling, dilated blood vessels, and petechiae of the soft and hard palate may occur (Damm and others, 1981; Elam, 1986; Schlesinger, Borbotsina, O'Neill, 1975) because of negative pressure produced in the posterior oropharynx (Belizzi, 1980).

Anal Findings

Of those who engage in anal intercourse, 50% have evident injury (Greene, 1996). Figure 2-30 shows the percentage of victims (*n* = 213) with anal or rectal injury compared with

genital injury. Serious injury is rare with penile penetration of the anus because the anus and anal canal are expansible and under voluntary control. Healing is rapid because of the rich blood supply, and injuries may be virtually undetectable by the untrained examiner 2 to 3 weeks postassault. Acute perianal TEARS are significant for sexual assault. More serious anal injuries may occur when no lubrication is used or with more forceful sexual practices such as the insertion of a hand, known as "fisting" (Wissow, 1992). Fisting has been associated with pelvic cellulitis. Perforation is more likely from inserting foreign objects. Anal scars may cross the dentate line. The scar tissue may disintegrate and form anal fissures.

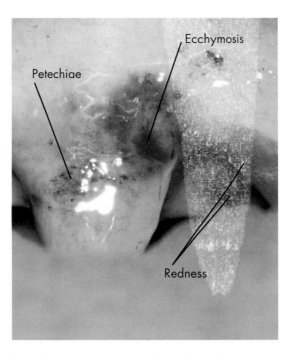

FIGURE 2-29 Ecchymosis and petechiae on the uvula (×15). There is redness on the left palatoglossal and palatopharyngeal arches with no redness on the corresponding right arches. This was associated with forced digital oral penetration. OUTCOME: Perpetrator is at large.

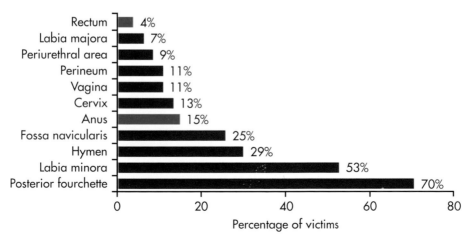

FIGURE 2-30 Location and frequency of injury in 213 sexually assaulted victims. (*From Slaughter and others*: *The pattern of genital injury in female sexual assault victims*, Am J Ob Gyn *176:609, 1997.*)

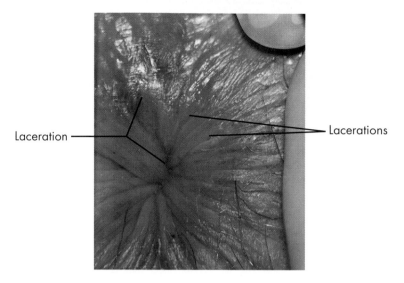

Laceration — Lacerations

FIGURE 2-31   Perianal lacerations and redness (×15). Lacerations are at 11 o'clock, 1 o'clock, and 2 o'clock. Redness is at 10 o'clock to 1 o'clock. The patient is a 24-year-old Hispanic female who was sodomized while kneeling, by an unidentified male.

Table 2-3 *Significant Nonspecific Perianal Findings*	
FINDINGS PROBABLY RELATED TO NONCONSENSUAL SEXUAL CONTACT	PERIANAL FINDINGS
Distorted irregular anal folds	Perianal skin tags
	Hyperpigmentation
Immediate (within 30 seconds) dilatation ≥ 20mm of the anus with no stool palpable or visible within rectal ampulla	Flat or thick anal folds at 6 o'clock and 12 o'clock
	Diastasis ani-smooth area of no folds at 6 o'clock and 12 o'clock
Flaccid rectal tone for first 12 to 48 hours postassault, resulting from damage to external sphincter	Anal fissures
Fixed opening of anus	Anal dilatation or opening of the external and internal anal sphincters as a result of feces in rectal ampulla
Rectal sphincter spasm	
Erythema and edema of the perianal tissue with pain and bleeding	Erythema
Perianal scar associated with an asymmetry in the shape of the anus when it is closed	Venous congestion causing local or diffuse discoloration
	Tightening or relaxing of anus when buttocks is spread
Perianal lacerations extending beyond the external anal sphincter	Pain on defecation
	Cellulitis
Semen retrieved from the anal canal	Hemorrhoids

Adapted from Adams JA, Knudson S: Genital findings in adolescent girls referred for suspected sexual abuse, *Arch Pediatr Adolescent Med* 150:850, 1996.

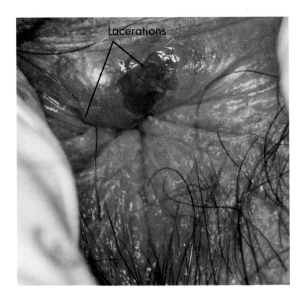

FIGURE 2-32 Perianal lacerations and redness (×15). Lacerations are at 10 o'clock and 12 o'clock. Redness is from 10 o'clock to 12 o'clock. This Samoan 14-year-old was sodomized by an unidentified male while she was bent over the sink. The examination was 4 hours postassault.

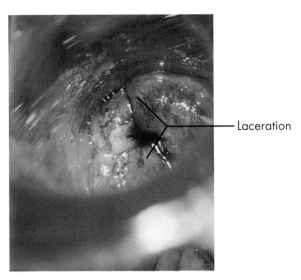

FIGURE 2-33 Anal mucosal laceration viewed through the end of an anoscope at 8 cm into the anal canal (×15). Injury was secondary to sodomy. Examination was 3 hours postassault.

Normal or nonspecific findings on anal examination do not rule out the possibility of nonconsensual sexual contact. Table 2-3 differentiates findings probably related to sexual assault from nonspecific perianal findings. The apex of delta-shaped abrasions or lacerations were once believed to point in the direction of the penetrating object. No clear data supports that understanding. Careful documentation of all findings should be made. Figures 2-31 and 2-32 are injuries of the perianal area. Figures 2-33 and 2-34 are injuries of the rectal mucosa.

Nongenital Findings

Nongenital injury has traditionally indicated resistance to perpetrator attacks and therefore that the incident was nonconsensual (Warner, Hewitt, 1993). Conversely, when there was no

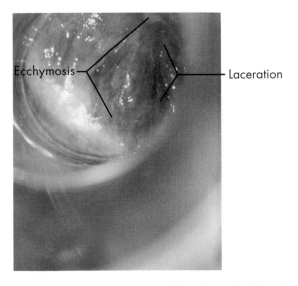

FIGURE 2-34 Rectal mucosal ecchymosis from 3 o'clock to 5 o'clock (×15). There is a vertical laceration 1 o'clock to 4 o'clock. The injury is secondary to sodomy and is viewed through an anoscope at 5 cm into the anal canal.

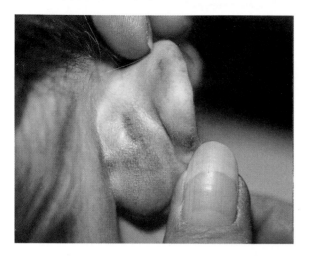

FIGURE 2-35 Ecchymosis on the posterior aspect of the pinna of the right ear (35mm). Ecchymosis is from forceful holding during nonconsensual oral copulation in this white 18-year-old female.

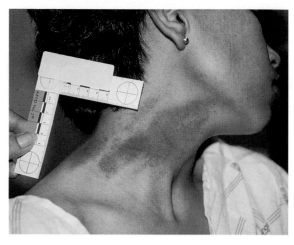

FIGURE 2-36 Right neck ecchymosis (35 mm). History revealed being held in a head lock from behind.

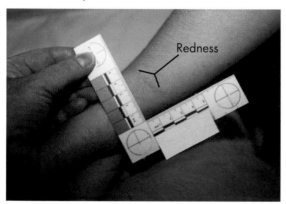

FIGURE 2-37 Redness on forearm from being tied with the patient's panty hose (35mm). Her arms were behind her back.

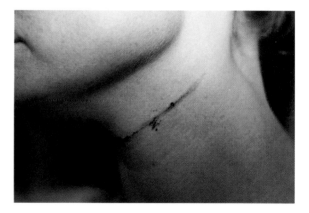

FIGURE 2-38 Cut to anterior neck (35mm). The patient stated the perpetrator cut her with a machete when she resisted him.

physical injury, the incident was believed to be consensual.

Nongenital trauma occurs in 30% to 45% of sexual assault patients. In more recent studies (Slaughter, 1997), the prevalence has increased, suggesting an increasing trend in violence. The presence of nongenital trauma is positively associated with genital trauma. Of sexually assaulted patients, 5% have major nongenital

physical injury, and one tenth of 1% die from asphyxiation and beating (Deming, Mittleman, Wetli, 1983). Although the elderly patient experiences physical force, extragenital trauma is less compared with the younger assaulted patient (Ramin and others, 1992).

Nongenital injury may be limited by the failure to resist. Victims may be unable to resist because of immobilizing fear that is present

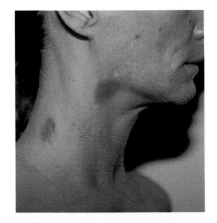

FIGURE 2-39 Ecchymosis to the right neck, two sites (35mm). The patient stated oral suction was applied to her neck.

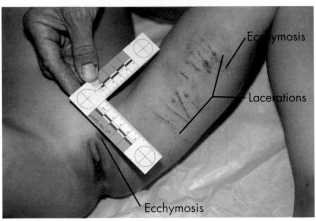

FIGURE 2-40 Linear-patterned injury (35mm). Lacerations and ecchymosis are on the inner aspect of the left thigh with ecchymosis at 1 o'clock on the left labium major. Her elongated clitoris is a variation not related to the assault. The patient, a Hispanic 8-year-old girl, Tanner Stage 1, physically and sexually abused by her stepfather, was brought to the United States for examination by a sexual assault expert. OUTCOME: Perpetrator was jailed in his country.

during the attack (Burgess, Fehder, Hartman, 1995). Furthermore, bruises may not have yet developed when the patient reports immediately for an examination. Bites of the face and breasts (Golden, 1996), suction injuries of neck and breasts, and grab marks on the arms and legs are the nongenital injuries that are commonly seen.

Injuries on the posterior auricle and to the tissue overlying the mastoid bone behind the ears may be caused by the perpetrator holding the victim for oral intercourse (Figure 2-35). These injuries may be called "clapping injuries." Figure 2-36 shows injuries from re-

straining the victim. Figure 2-37 shows injuries from restraints applied to the wrists. A machete cut of the anterior neck, inflicted while abducting the patient, is shown in Figure 2-38. The ecchymosis in Figure 2-39 is from suction. Figure 2-40 shows patterned laceration and bruising from keys on the belt of the perpetrator. Figures 2-41 to 2-44 are bite marks. Photographs or castings of bite marks and the saliva obtained from swabbing bite marks may be critical in identifying the perpetrator. Casting bite marks requires special training based on a standard protocol from the American Society of Forensic Odontology (ASFO).

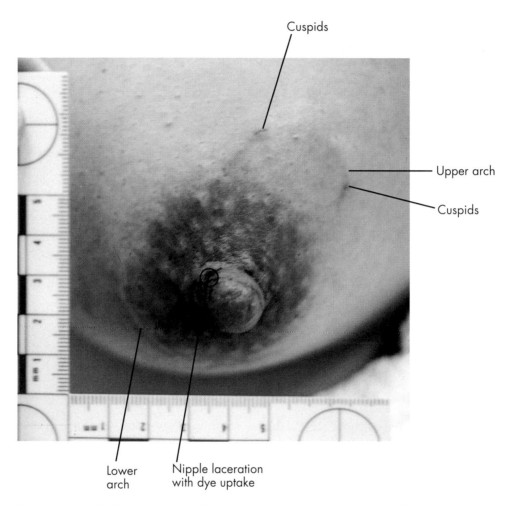

Cuspids

Upper arch

Cuspids

Lower arch

Nipple laceration with dye uptake

FIGURE 2-41 Left breast bite mark and nipple laceration (35mm). The bite mark is three dimensional (length, width, and depth). Depth or indentation in the upper arch is from the cuspids. The depth of the injury is evident clinically, but not captured well in the photograph. Lacerations to the medial aspect of the left nipple are highlighted with Toluidine Blue dye (35mm). This Asian 37 year old also experienced penile vaginal penetration.

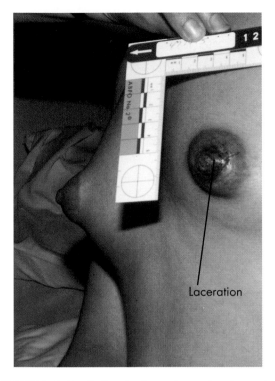

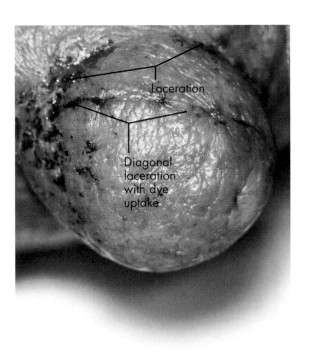

FIGURE 2-42 Left nipple and areolar laceration (35mm) . History revealed this was secondary to suction bites in this white 16 year old.

FIGURE 2-43 Nipple lacerations (×15), showing Toluidine Blue dye uptake at 9 o'clock to 12 o'clock, and 1 o'clock to 2 o'clock, as well as diagonally across the nipple from 10 o'clock to 3 o'clock. The nipple lacerations are consistent with the history of suction and bites to the breast.

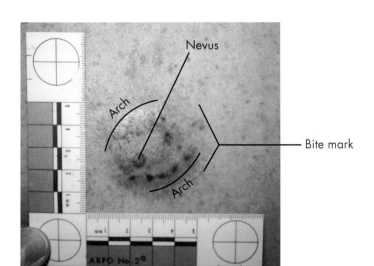

FIGURE 2-44 Three-dimensional bite mark on the back (length, width, and depth) (35mm). Patient is a male 31 year old whose girlfriend bit him on his back through his T-shirt.

Case Findings in Female Sexual Assault: Adult, Adolescent, and Elderly

Case One: This 22-year-old, sexually active, Caucasian female (Figures 2-45 to 2-49) was at the beach with a female friend when she was abducted by three unknown males, one African American and two Caucasians. She was taken to the car. Over the course of several hours, two of the males repeatedly penetrated her vagina and anus with their fingers and penises, while the third male continued driving. She was positioned supine and kneeling, during the assaults in the backseat of the car. In a remote canyon, the perpetrators "dumped [her] out of the car" and "pushed [her] down a hillside." Her sexual assault examination with colposcopy was conducted 2 hours after she was released from the perpetrators. The findings supported the history of the reported incident. After several months the driver reported the incident. A military court-martial sentenced all three perpetrators to military prison. One received life in prison, another received 40 years, and the driver was sentenced to 3 years in prison.

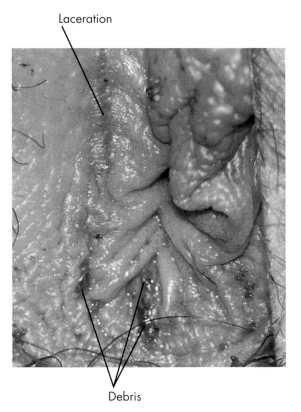

Laceration

Debris

FIGURE 2-45 Laceration to the right labium major (×15). Sand and debris are present. Genitalia are acutely tender by history.

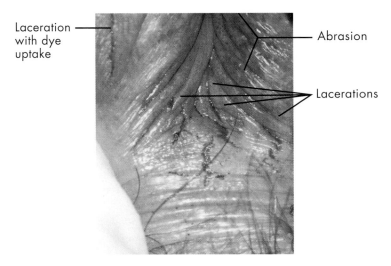

Laceration with dye uptake

Abrasion

Lacerations

FIGURE 2-46 Labium major and multiple posterior fourchette lacerations (×15). Toluidine Blue dye uptake is patchy, since lacerations are still oozing at 3 hours postassault. An abrasion is present on the left labium minor.

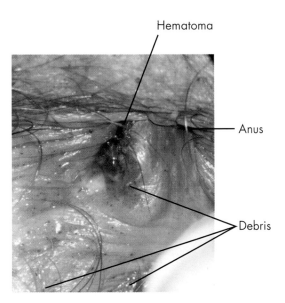

Hematoma

Anus

Debris

FIGURE 2-47 Perianal hematoma (×15). Hematoma is at 8 o'clock to 9 o'clock with perianal redness. Particles of sand and debris are present in perianal area.

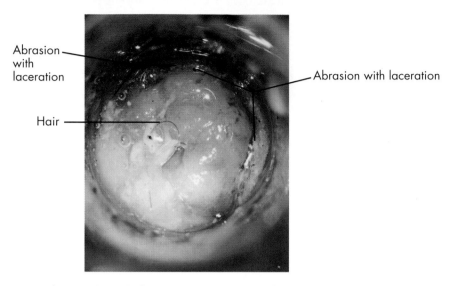

Abrasion with laceration

Abrasion with laceration

Hair

FIGURE 2-48 Anal canal abrasions and lacerations from 10 o'clock to 3 o'clock. Several black debris particles are present and a hair is present centrally. The bluish color from 3 o'clock to 5 o'clock at the rim and outside the anoscope need to be further evaluated by repositioning the anoscope.

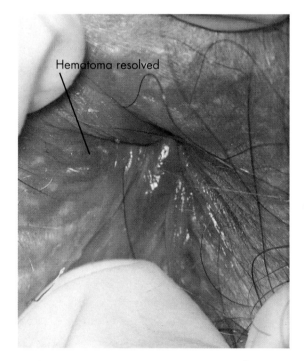

Hematoma resolved

FIGURE 2-49 Perianal healing (×15). Patient was rechecked 14 days postassault. Hematoma has resolved. Some residual swelling and redness is present. The patient denied pain in passing stool.

Case Two: A 15-year-old "sexually active," Caucasian female was assaulted on a bed in the supine position (Figures 2-50 to 2-53). The perpetrator was a 22-year-old acquaintance who gave her a ride home from school. She was vaginally penetrated "several times" alternately, with his fingers and penis. She arrived 3 hours postassault for a medical-legal examination.

Although she admitted to being sexually active, she repeatedly asked during the examination, "Am I still a virgin?" This is a common question for adolescents. The examiner determined from further exploration that the patient was asking two questions: "Is my hymen still present?" and "What is a virgin?" The examiner described the injury that was present and affirmed that her hymen was still present. The dictionary definition of "virgin" was explained. The history was confirmed by a jury conviction for rape with an underage victim.

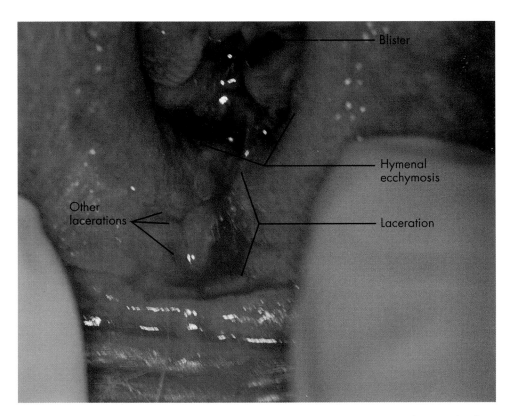

FIGURE 2-50   Posterior fourchette laceration (×15). Large laceration extends into the fossa navicularis. There are other fourchette lacerations. Hymenal ecchymosis extends from 5 o'clock to 8 o'clock and a blood- and fluid-filled blister is present at 3 o'clock. Labia minora are red and swollen. There has been no Toluidine Blue dye applied. The injuries were obvious before this magnified view.

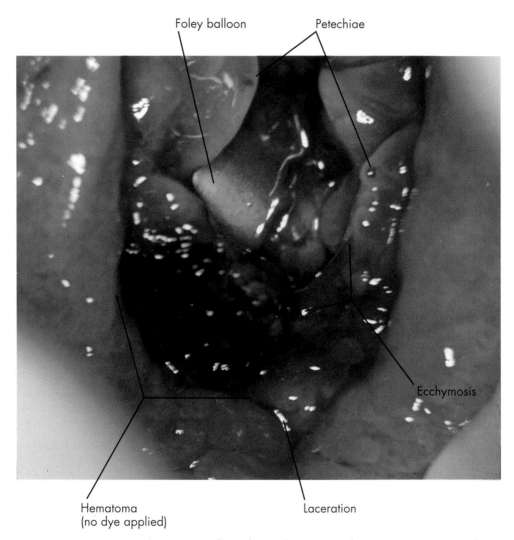

Foley balloon   Petechiae

Ecchymosis

Hematoma
(no dye applied)   Laceration

FIGURE 2-51 Hymenal hematoma from 6 o'clock to 8 o'clock (×15). There is an inflated Foley catheter balloon just distal to the hymen, which straightens the hymenal folds and helps demonstrate the hematoma. Ecchymosis is present from 4 o'clock to 6 o'clock with petechiae on the hymen. The labia minora are red with lacerations on their inferior ends.

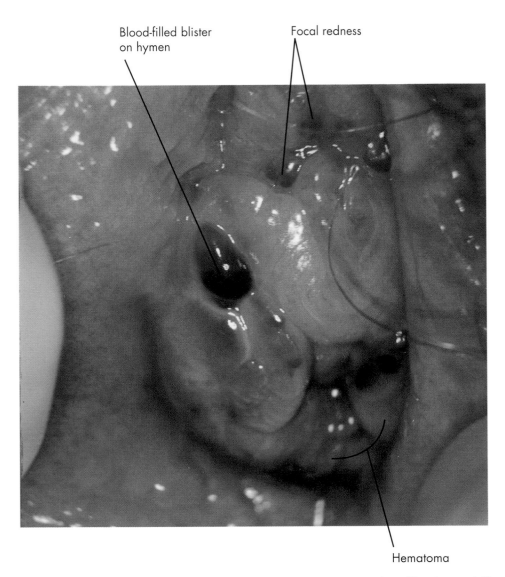

Blood-filled blister on hymen

Focal redness

Hematoma

FIGURE 2-52   Blood-and-fluid-filled blister on hymen (×15). Hymenal swelling is especially present from 12 o'clock to 2 o'clock with focal areas of redness at 12 o'clock to 1 o'clock. Hymenal hematoma at 3 o'clock to 8 o'clock, which is also shown at another angle in Figure 2-51.

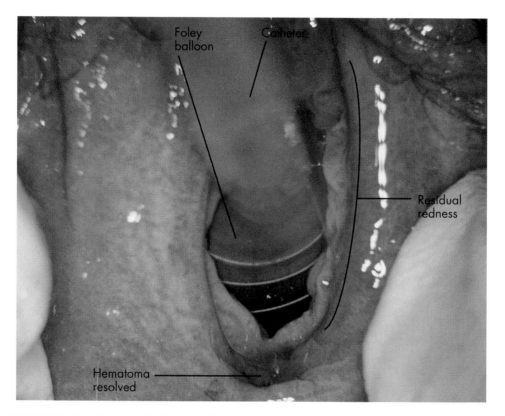

FIGURE 2-53 Hymenal healing, 16 days postassault (×15). The hematoma has resolved, but there is Toluidine Blue dye uptake at the site of the healing hematoma, and the left labium minor is red. A Foley catheter balloon is in the vaginal orifice.

Case Three: A Caucasian 73-year-old female was awakened from sleep in her home to find her neighbor's son on top of her (Figures 2-54 to 2-57). She was examined within 8 hours of the assault. She was penetrated vaginally with his finger and said, "I don't know how many times. He looked wild and I screamed, but it didn't help." The findings of the medical-legal examination supported the history and timing of the reported incident. The history was confirmed by a jury conviction for rape with a foreign object and abuse of the elderly. He was sentenced to 25 years to life in prison.

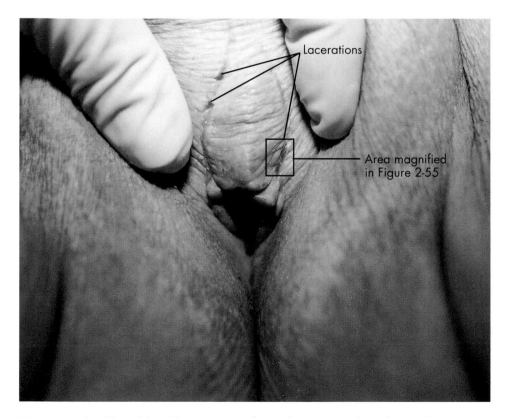

FIGURE 2-54   Clitoral hood lacerations at 4 o'clock , 10 o'clock, and 11 o'clock (35mm). There is also swelling of the clitoral hood, evident when compared with the follow-up photograph (see Figure 2-57). She is 30 years posthysterectomy and is not taking estrogen. The sagging tissue and lack of pubic hair are characteristics of the elderly.

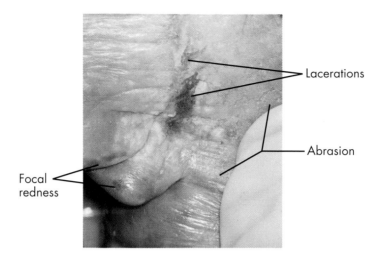

FIGURE 2-55 Clitoral hood laceration (×15). This is the laceration on the left clitoral hood from Figure 2-54 seen here with magnification. Lateral to the laceration is an abrasion. Inferior to the laceration are focal areas of redness.

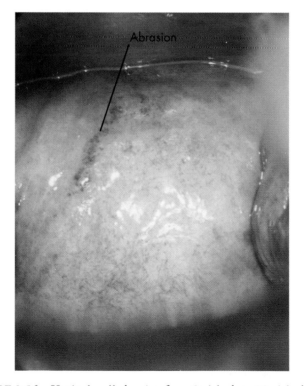

FIGURE 2-56 Vaginal wall abrasion from 9 o'clock to 12 o'clock (×15).

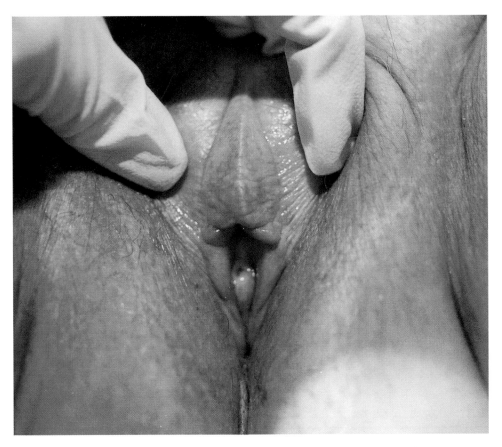

FIGURE 2-57   Clitoral hood healing (35mm). Follow-up examination is 6 months post-assault. Lacerations are healed (35mm).

FINDINGS IN THE ASSAULTED MALE: ADULT AND ADOLESCENT

Incidence and Factors Related to Male Sexual Assault

Males report 48,500 sexual assaults per year, that is, 0.5 reports of sexual assault per 1,000 persons age 12 or older (Bureau of Justice Statistics, 1995a). When the perpetrator is a family member, the mean age for victimization of males is 11 years. Hillman (1990) studied 100 males who were accessed from a sexual assault counseling center. These males were initially assaulted at 14.5 years (with a range of 3 to 43 years). The mean age at presentation for counseling was 25.3 years. When the male patient is a homosexual, the mean age of assault is approximately 22 years (with a range of 15 to 57 years). Of homosexual men, 28% report being sexually assaulted in their lifetime (Hickson and others, 1994).

In Hillman's study (1990) the perpetrator was known by the patient in 72% of the cases and was a family member in 28% of the cases. Of the patients, 75% were assaulted on more than one occasion, and 43% reported multiple perpetrators. Female perpetrators were rare and if present, were accompanied by male perpetrators (Hillman, 1990). Hickson and others (1994) found that of 930 homosexual patients, 3.9% of the perpetrators were female.

Use of weapons and brutality were reported more often with male sexually assaulted patients (Hillman, 1990). Males sustain more physical trauma and are held captive longer than females (Kaufman and others, 1980). Male-on-male attacks were often gang-related, motivated by the need to assert power, release aggression, and control feelings of hopelessness (McMullen, 1990). Twenty percent reported that the perpetrator claimed to be infected with the human immunodeficiency virus (HIV) (Hillman, 1990). Most male patients reported that they felt their lives were in danger at the time of the assault.

The most common forms of sexual assault in males were receptive anal intercourse (75%), forced manual genital stimulation of the assailant (65%), receptive oral intercourse (59%), and forced manual genital stimulation of the patient (55%). More than half of the males experienced more than one type of nonconsensual sexual contact (Hillman, 1990). Some men experience an erection and/or ejaculation during the assault, but both of these responses can occur as involuntary reactions to extreme stress and may be purely physiological. A male does not have to be sexually aroused to have an erection (Oakleaf, 1996). In Hillman's study (1990), 33 of 100 males experienced disruption of skin or mucous membranes related to the assault. In another study (Hillman and others, 1991) of 28 male victims with a mean age of assault of 21.7 years, 89% sustained penetrative anal intercourse, and 57% had skin or mucosal injury.

More than half of the 100 males evidenced STDs at the time of the examination, which patients attributed to the assault. About half of the patients reported they were homosexuals (Hillman, 1990). In a second study of male sexually assaulted victims ($n = 28$) conducted by retrospective chart review, Hillman and others (1991) found STDs in 18%. The STDs were presumed secondary to the assault.

Only 12% of men reported the sexual assault to the police, and another 12% reported it to medical personnel. Of those reporting to medical personnel, more reported to family physicians than to emergency department staff. Males report victimization less often than females. Explanations include the stigma of presumed homosexuality, the perceived insensitivity to homosexuality by law enforcement and health care providers toward homosexuality, and the humiliation of being used sexually by another male (McMullen, 1990). Their masculinity is further threatened because they were not able to defend themselves.

When a male arrives at the emergency department with injuries from physical assault, especially at the hands of multiple perpetrators or when a deadly weapon was used, the possibility of sexual assault should be considered.

CASE FINDINGS IN MALE SEXUAL ASSAULT: ADULT AND ADOLESCENT

Case One: A 28-year-old Hispanic male was beaten up at a party he was attending (Figures 2-58 and 2-59). A bottle of beer was put up his anus. He reported for the examination, 12 hours postassault. The findings were consistent with the history and timing of the reported incident. The patient left the country instead of appearing for court.

Lacerations

Lacerations

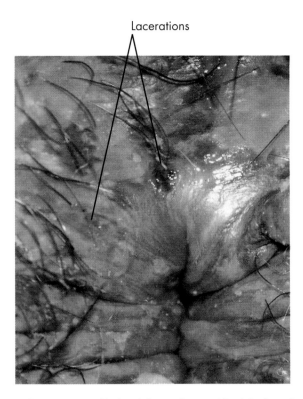

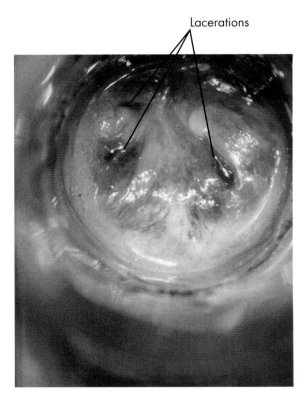

FIGURE 2-58   Perianal laceration at 10 o'clock and 12 o'clock (×15). There is swelling, evident by the smoothness of the perianal folds, especially from 10 o'clock to 2 o'clock in contrast to the folds present from 2 o'clock to 10 o'clock. Grey areas are pigmentation and not ecchymosis.

FIGURE 2-59   Rectal mucosal lacerations (×15). Lacerations are present at 4 o'clock, 9 o'clock, and 10 o'clock as viewed through an anoscope at 5 cm into the anal canal. Swelling and redness are throughout.

Case Two: A 15-year-old African-American male was beaten and sexually assaulted by a group of five "family members and friends" in their living room (Figures 2-60 to 2-62). The adolescent perpetrators held the 15-year-old bent over the sofa. The female leader of the group of four adolescents digitally penetrated the anus of the 15 year old. She put a condom on a 6-inch rubber dildo, lubricated it with cocoa butter, and inserted it in his anus. Before and after the anal assault, the 15 year old was hit with fists in the face and was beaten "all over my body" with a mop handle and belt buckle. The patient ran away; the case was dropped.

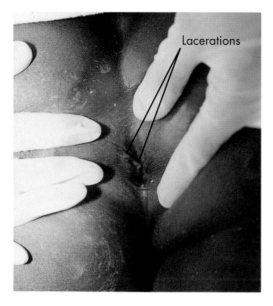

FIGURE 2-60   Perianal lacerations at 11 o'clock and 12 o'clock viewed without magnification (35mm).

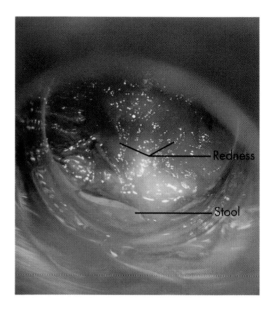

FIGURE 2-61   Reddened anal mucosa viewed through an anoscope at 5 cm (×15).

FIGURE 2-62   Ecchymosis of the lower lip with surrounding redness (35mm). Abrasion on the tongue and a laceration of the upper lip is from being "punched in the face."

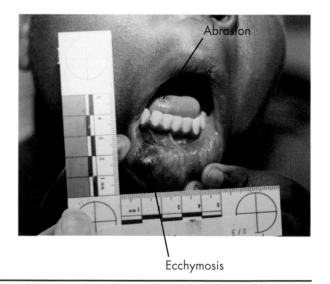

FINDINGS IN CONSENSUAL INTERCOURSE

Injury is unusual in consensual intercourse. Slaughter (1997) found in her group of consenting volunteers ($n = 75$) that injury occurred in 11% compared with injury in 89% of the sexually assaulted patients ($n = 311$). The sites of injury are the same as in nonconsensual intercourse, but the number of sites injured per person was less in the volunteers having consensual intercourse than in those who were assaulted. The absence of the normal sexual response may explain the injury that occurs in consensual intercourse, because when superficial lacerations have been found, there is a history of dry and painful consensual intercourse (Lauber, Souma, 1982; Paul, 1977).

After consensual intercourse, 4% (Lauber, Souma, 1982) to 10% (McCauley and others, 1987) of adult women had posterior fourchette lacerations, which were detected without magnification. Sexually assaulted patients were 16 times more likely to have lacerations confirmed by the uptake of Toluidine Blue dye (McCauley and others, 1987) as compared with volunteers following consensual intercourse. Multiparity is associated with less injury because of the greater flexibility or distensibility of the introitus.

Hypervascularity is not considered to be traumatic nor a blunt force of trauma. Hypervascularity of the vaginal mucosa was the most consistent finding after consensual intercourse ($n = 17$) according to Norvell, Benrubi, and Thompson (1984). They focused on vaginal changes in consenting intercourse, using magnification. They did not report the findings on the external genitalia. The etiologic factors of the hypervascularity were not determined, but it may be a normal variant or a result of normal physiological changes because it has also been identified before intercourse. Figures 2-63 to 2-66 show examples of findings associated with consensual intercourse.

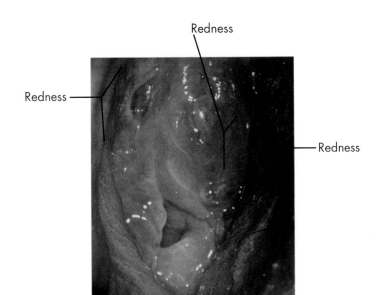

Redness

Redness

Redness

FIGURE 2-63 Consensual findings (Figures 2-63 to 2-66). Hymen and left labium minor redness (×15). Redness is from 2 o'clock to 4 o'clock and 7 o'clock to 10 o'clock on the hymen and 2 o'clock to 6 o'clock on the left labium minor, 3 hours after consensual intercourse. The patient was positioned supine and side-lying during the intercourse.

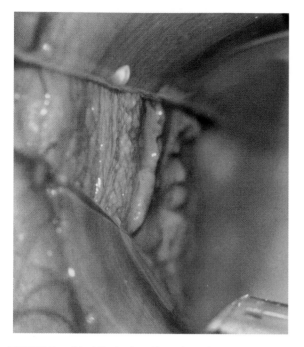

FIGURE 2-64 Vaginal wall, pink and unswollen, free of TEARS (×15).

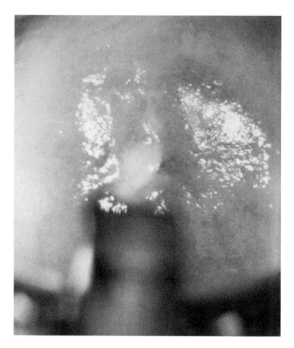

FIGURE 2-65 Cervix, before consensual intercourse, pink and free of TEARS (×15).

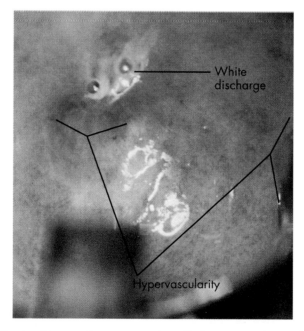

FIGURE 2-66 Cervix, 4 hours after consensual penile intercourse (×15). Compare with Figure 2-65, before intercourse. There is hypervascularity at 12 o'clock and 3 o'clock, and in the quadrant from 12 o'clock to 3 o'clock.

Slaughter (1997) found local or general hypervascularity on the external or internal genitalia (Figure 2-66). Six volunteers of the 11% still had hypervascularity at follow-up. Hypervascularity may be a persistent finding in some females and in the same posterior locations as that seen with nonconsensual intercourse, including the posterior fourchette, labia minora, hymen and fossa navicularis (see Table 2-2) but the persistence is less.

In adolescents ages 12 to 18, the incidence of perineal lacerations in consensual intercourse was similar to that in sexual assault. The similar prevalence between consenting and nonconsenting intercourse was explained by the spasticity of the pubococcygeus muscle (McCauley, Gorman, Guzinski, 1987). Therefore consent does not preclude trauma in adults or in adolescents but the prevalence of injury is less than in those who have been sexually assaulted.

REFERENCES

Adams JA, Knudson S: Genital findings in adolescent girls referred for suspected sexual abuse, *Arch Pediatr Adolescent Med* 150:850, 1996.

Aiken MM: False allegation: a concept in the context of rape, *J Psychosoc Nur* 31:15, 1993.

Battiste-Otto F: *Personal communication,* March, 1996.

Bellizzi R, Krakow AM, Plack W: Soft palate trauma associated with fellatio, *Mil Med* 145:787, 1980.

Brauner P, Gallili N: A condom the critical link in a rape, *J Forensic Sci* 38: 1233, 1993.

Bureau of Justice Statistics: *National crime victimization survey: preliminary results for 1995,* Washington, DC, 1996, US Department of Justice.

Bureau of Justice Statistics: *Violent crime* (NCJ-147486), Washington, DC, 1995a, US Department of Justice.

Bureau of Justice Statistics: *Violence against women: Estimates from the redesigned survey* (NCJ-154348), Washington, DC, 1995b, US Department of Justice.

Bureau of Justice Statistics: *Elderly crime victims* (NCJ-147186), Washington, DC, 1994, US Department of Justice.

Burgess AW, Fehder W, Hartman CR: Delayed reporting of the rape victim, *J Psychosoc Nur* 33:21, 1995.

Cartwright P, Moore, A: Elderly victims of rape, *South Med J* 82:988, 1989.

Cartwright PS: Factors that correlate with injury sustained by survivors of sexual assault, *Ob Gyn* 70:44, 1987.

Centers for Disease Control and Prevention: *Sexually transmitted disease treatment guidelines, MMWR,* No RR-14, 42:1993.

Crowley S: *Sexual assault statistics.* Paper presented at Sexual Assault Examiner Training Course in Palm Springs, Calif, March 1996.

Damm D, White D, Brinker M: (1981). Variations of palatal erythema secondary to fellatio, *Oral Surg* 52:417, 1981.

Davis TC, Peck GQ, Storment JM: Acquaintance rape and the high school student, *J Adolesc Health* 14:220, 1993.

Deming JE, Mittleman RE, Wetli CV: Forensic science aspects of fatal sexual assaults on women, *J Forensic Sci* 28:572, 1983.

Douglas JE and others: *Crime classification manual,* New York, 1992, MacMillan.

Draucker CB: *The victimization of sexual abuse survivors in adulthood,* unpublished manuscript, Kent State University, 1996.

Elam AL, Ray VG: Sexually related trauma: a review, *Ann Emerg Med* 15:576, 1986.

Federal Bureau of Investigation: *Uniform crime reports for the United States, 1992,* Washington, DC, 1993, US Department of Justice.

Feldman MD, Ford CV, Stone T: Deceiving others/deceiving oneself: 4 cases of factitious rape, *South Med J* 87:736, 1994.

Frieze IH, Browne A: Violence in marriage. In Ohlin L, Tonry M, editors: *Family violence: crime and justice, a review of research,* Chicago, 1989, University of Chicago Press.

Geist RF: Sexually related trauma, *Emerg Med Clin No Am* 6:439, 1988.

Gibbons M, Vincent E: Childhood sexual abuse, *Amer Fam Phys* 49:1, 1994.

Golden G: *Forensic odontology.* Paper presented at Sexual Assault Examiner Training Course in Palm Springs, Calif, March 1996.

Graves HCB, Sensabaugh GF, Blake ET: Postcoital detection of a male-specific semen protein: application to the investigation of rape, *N Engl J Med* 312:1735, 1985.

Greene, J: Genital-Anal trauma secondary to sexual assault. Paper presented at the US Naval Hospital, San Diego, January 1996.

Groth, AN: *Men who rape,* New York, 1979, Plenum Press.

Groth AN, Burgess AW: Sexual dysfunction during rape, *N Engl J Med* 297:764, 1977.

Heger A, Emans SJ: *Evaluation of the sexually abused child,* New York, 1992, Oxford.

Hibbard RA, Ingersoll GM, Orr DP: Behavioral risk and child abuse among adolescents in a nonclinical setting, *Pediatrics* 86:896, 1990.

Hickson GCI and others: Gay men as victims of nonconsensual sex, *Arch Sex Behav* 23:281, 1994.

Hillman R: Medical and social aspects of sexual assault of males: a survey of 100 victims, *Brit J Gen Pract* 40:502, 1990.

Hillman R and others: Adult male victims of sexual assault: an underdiagnosed condition, *Int J STD AIDS* 2:22, 1991.

Jenny C and others: Sexually transmitted diseases in victims of rape, *N Engl J Med* 322:713, 1990.

Kaufman A and others: Male rape: noninstitutionalized assault, *Am J Psychiat* 137:221, 1980.

Koss MP: Hidden rape: sexual aggression and victimization in a national sample of students in higher education. In Burgess, AW, editor: *Rape and sexual assault,* New York, 1988, Garland.

Koss MP, Dinero TE, Seibel CA: Stranger and acquaintance rape: are there differences in the victim's experience? *Psychol Wom Quar* 12:1, 1988.

Lauber AA, Souma, ML: Use of toluidine blue for documentation of traumatic intercourse, *Ob Gyn* 60:644, 1982.

McCall GJ: Risk factors for sexual assault prevention, *J Interpersonal Viol* 8:277, 1993.

McCauley J, Gorman RL, Guzinski G: Toluidine blue in the detection of perineal lacerations in pediatric and adolescent sexual abuse victims, *Pediatrics* 78:1039, 1986.

McMullen R: *Male rape: breaking the silence on the last taboo,* London, 1990, Gay Men's Press.

Nagy S, Adcock AG, Nagy MC: A comparison of health risk behaviors of sexually active sexually abused and abstaining adolescents, *Pediatrics* 93:570, 1994.

Norvell MK, Benrubi, GI Thompson RJ: Investigation of microtrauma after sexual intercourse, *J Reprod Med* 29:269, 1984.

Oakleaf L: *Men and sexual assault,* March 1996. Online address: loakleaf@midway.uchicago.edu

Office of Criminal Justice: *California medical protocol for examination of sexual assault and child sexual abuse victims,* Sacramento, 1987, author.

Paul D: The medical examination of the live rape victim and the accused, *Leg Med Ann* 139, 1977.

Rambow B, Atkinson C, Frost TH and others: Female sexual assault medical and legal implications, *Ann Emerg Med* 21:727, 1992.

Ramin SM, and others: Sexual assault in postmenopausal women, *Ob Gyn* 80:86, 1992.

Rapaport KR, Posey CD: Sexually coercive college males. In Parrot A, editor, *Acquaintance rape: the hidden crime,* New York, 1991, John Wiley.

Rupp JC: Sperm survival and prostatic acid phosphatase activity in victims of sexual assault, *J Forens Sci* 14:177, 1969.

Satin AJ and others: Sexual assault in pregnancy, *Ob Gyn* 77:710, 1991.

Schlesinger SL, Borbotsina J, O'Neill L: Petechial hemorrhages of the soft palate secondary to fellatio, *Oral Surg* 40:376, 1976.

Secofsky S: *The crime lab.* Paper presented at Sexual Assault Examiner Training Course in Palm Springs, Calif, March, 1996.

Seneski P: *Sexual assault in the elderly.* Paper presented at Examiner Training Course in Palm Springs, Calif, March, 1996.

Slaughter L and others: The pattern of genital injury in female sexual assault victims, *Am J Ob Gyn* 176:609, 1997.

Slaughter L: *Personal communication,* December, 1996.

Slaughter L, Brown CRV: Colposcopy to establish physical findings in rape victims, *Am J Ob Gyn* 166:83, 1992.

Slaughter L, Brown CRV: Cervical findings in rape victims, *Am J Ob Gyn* 164:528, 1991.

Slaughter L, Crowley S: Prevalence of sexually transmitted diseases in sex offenders. Paper presented at North American Association of Pediatric and Adolescent Gynecology, April 1993.

Slaughter L, Shackleford S: Genital injury in rape, *Adolesc Pediatr Gynecol* 6:175, 1993.

Sorenson SB, Siegel JN, Golding JN: Repeated sexual victimization, *Violence and Victims* 6:299, 1991.

Tyra P: Older women: victims of rape, *J Geriatr Nurs* 19:7, 1993.

US Department of Commerce: *Statistical abstract of the United States, 1994,* Washington, DC, 1994, Economics and Statistics Administration.

Warner A, Hewitt J: Victim resistance and judgments of victim consensuality in rape (3 pt 1), *Percept Mot Skills* 76:952, 1993

White J, Humphrey JA: Young people's attitudes toward acquaintance rape, In *Acquaintance rape: the hidden crime,* New York, 1991, John Wiley.

Wissow LS: Child sexual abuse. In Carpenter JA, editor: *Pediatric and adolescent gynecology,* New York, 1992, Raven.

SUGGESTED READINGS

Ageton SS: *Sexual assault among adolescents,* Lexington, Mass, 1983, Heath.

Committee of Adolescence: Sexual assault and the adolescent, *Pediatrics* 94:761, 1994.

Hillman RJ, Tomlinson D, McMillan A and others: Sexual assault of men: a series, *Genitourin Med* 66:247, 1990.

Muram D, Miller K, Cutler A: Sexual assault of the elderly victim, *J of Interpers Viol* 7:70, 1992.

Scott CS, Lefley HP, Hick D: Potential risk factors for rape in three ethnic groups, *Comm Ment Health J* 29:133, 1993.

WEBSITES

The Bureau of Justice Statistics webpage address: http://www.ojp.usdoj.gov/bjs/

The California Criminalistics Institute (CCI) address: http://www.ns.net/cci

CCI is a leading postgraduate school for criminalists, a section of the California Department of Justice, Bureau of Forensic Services. The homepage contains course and class descriptions, and other information.

3 FINDINGS THAT RESULT FROM NONASSAULT INJURY, INFECTION, & OTHER NONASSAULT VARIATIONS

NONASSAULT INJURY

Alternative explanations for TEARS must be considered in patients reporting for a sexual assault examination. The history may identify these alternative explanations. The examiner must ask specifically about the possibilities for foreign object penetration, straddle injury, and/or sudden abduction of the lower extremities. The follow-up examination at 2 weeks after the initial examination also helps to differentiate physical findings, resulting from traumatic, nontraumatic, or other etiologic factors. Most acute injury heals at 2 weeks and scars may be the only evidence of a laceration. Therefore the comparison of the initial findings with findings from the follow-up examination is an important part of the care of the patient.

Vaginal penetration may occur from accidentally falling on objects or intentionally exploring orifices with an object. Accidental penetration from projections such as a picket fence or bike seat post may cause hymenal and vaginal injury. Ecchymotic areas could result from blunt objects or a puncture or cut from sharper objects. Intentional penetration in the prepubescent female is uncommon because the nonestrogenized hymen is quite sensitive and

voluntary exploration is painful. Self-penetration of the vagina in the prepubescent female is a good indication that sexual abuse may be occurring (Heger, 1996). In the pubescent female, self-penetration is more likely because of the onset of menses, the use of feminine hygiene products, and the nonpainful hymen.

Plastic applicators encasing the tampon may cause lacerations (Gray, Norton, and Treadwell, 1980), as indicated in Figures 3-1 and 3-2. Inserting tampons can also cause mechanical erosion (Danielson, 1983). However there is no data to support that tampon use causes hymenal injuries consistent with nonconsensual penetration injuries (Bays and others, 1990).

Retained vaginal foreign body such as a tampon may be detected when there is purulent or bloody discharge (Dudgeon, Paidas, 1992). Figure 3-3 shows cervical swelling and drying from a tampon retained for 3 days, or since the stated time of the assault. The 22-year-old patient reported for medical care because of the foul odor and discharge from her vagina. On speculum examination a tampon was located against the cervix, at the site of swelling. Friedrich and Siegesmund (1980) explained that tampon-associated mucosal drying and loss

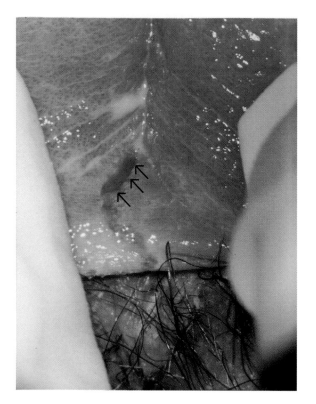

FIGURE 3-1 Tampon injury (Figures 3-1 to 3-3). Acute laceration (×15). Figures 3-1 and 3-2 are the same patient. The laceration is on the posterior fourchette at 6 o'clock in this sexually active, white, 15 year old. The laceration is visible without magnification. The patient said she inserted a plastic encased tampon 4 hours earlier and "it hurt when I put it in." Friable tissue from an ongoing yeast infection is prone to laceration injury from the plastic tampon applicator.

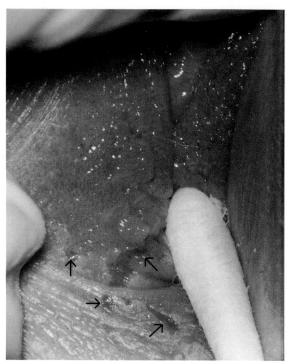

FIGURE 3-2 Tampon lacerations (×15). Other lacerations are evident by separating the tissue.

of cell coherence could occur from the superabsorbents when tampons were worn at times other than during active menstruation. Danielson (1983) explained that the synthetic cellulose acetate from which superabsorbents are made may become implanted in the vaginal mucosa and result in inflammation.

Fingers or fingernails (Figure 3-4), other foreign objects and even improperly handled vaginal specula (Figures 3-5 and 3-6) may also cause

genital injury (Lauber, Souma, 1982).

A straddle fall onto a horizontal bar of playground equipment or bicycle cross bar may appear as a minor laceration or abrasion with swelling and ecchymosis of the perineum, as well as the labia majora and minora. The mons, clitoris, and urethra may also be involved. More external injury often occurs than internal trauma (Gibbons, Vincent 1994). Straddle injuries occur most typically in 2-to-6 year olds (Berenson, 1996; Dudgeon, Paidas, 1992), but may occur in adolescents and adults.

Sudden abduction of the legs, which occurs in gymnastics, may cause vaginal orifice lacerations. Pelvic fractures involving hip joint disruption or resulting in sharp bony fragments

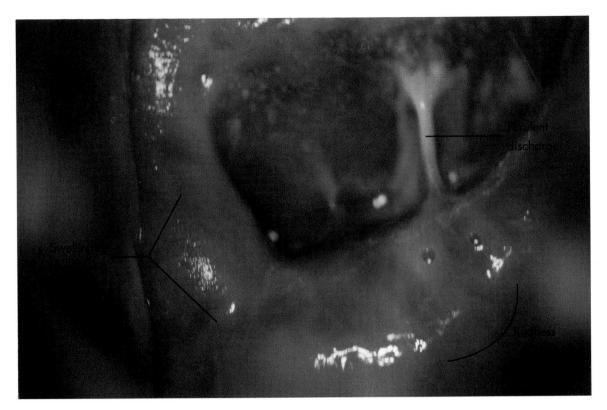

FIGURE 3-3 Cervical swelling and drying at 8 o'clock to 9 o'clock. The tampon was retrieved from that site and had been retained for 3 days in this 22 year old. Redness is apparent around the cervical os and at 6 o'clock.

may cause vaginal lacerations. However the incidence of such injuries is rare (Dudgeon, Paidas, 1992).

INFECTIONS

Sexually transmitted infection occurs as a result of rape in 4% to 30% of patients (Murphy, 1990). However sexually transmitted diseases (STDs) that are evident within 72 hours of the assault probably antedate the assault.

Jenny and others (1990) found STDs in 43% of 204 postmenarcheal girls and women exam-

ined within 72 hours postpenile vaginal assault. Patients were excluded if they were assaulted by a regular sexual partner or were victims of incest. Table 3-1 lists the STDs present at the initial examination and the risk of acquiring STDs. The risk was calculated at the follow-up examination, which was an average of 2.6 weeks from the first visit.

The infections most commonly diagnosed among women after sexual assault are trichomoniasis, chlamydia, gonorrhea, and bacterial vaginosis (Centers for Disease Control and

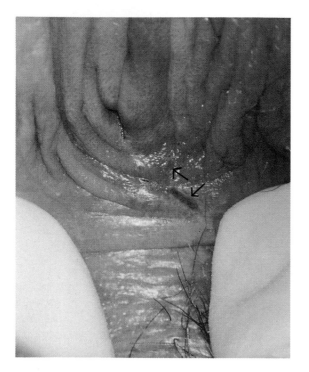

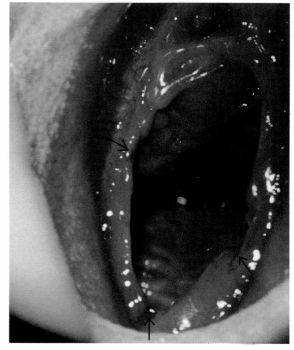

FIGURE 3-4 Fingernail laceration on the posterior fourchette at 5 o'clock (×15). The patient stated here at follow-up that she was feeling itchy and scratched herself there. She started over-the-counter intravaginal treatment for the yeast infection 24 hours before this examination and denies itching at the time of the photograph. OUTCOME: The case was dropped by the district attorney because the patient changed her story, and there was evidence to suggest that the reported assault was consensual intercourse.

FIGURE 3-5 Speculum injury (Figures 3-5 and 3-6). Healing lacerations of the hymen at 4 o'clock, 7 o'-clock, and 10 o'clock with general vulvular redness on this white 7 year old (×15). Figure 3-6 is of the same patient. This photograph was taken under anesthesia in the supine position, 72 hours postspeculum injury. The speculum examination was attempted for complaints of blood on the underwear. The child was expectedly uncooperative during the attempted speculum examination because of the sensitivity of the unestrogenized hymen. The history did not affirm that sexual assault had occurred. The cause for the blood was also not

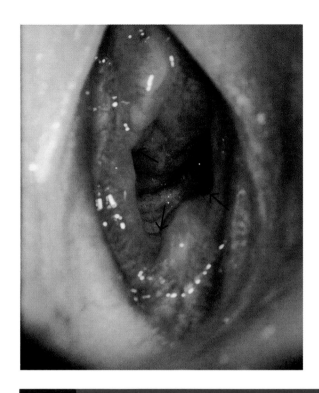

FIGURE 3-6 Healing hymenal lacerations (×15). Seven days after the initial injury, during this clinical examination, the lacerations at 4 o'clock, 7 o'clock, and 10 o'clock are significantly healed. Redness is reduced. There was no long-term follow-up to determine the hymenal configuration after healing.

Table 3-1	*Sexually Transmitted Diseases at Initial Examination and Follow-Up*	
STD ORGANISMS	PERCENT AT 72 HOURS	PERCENT RISK OF ACQUIRING*
Bacterial vaginosis (anaerobes, *Gardnerella vaginalis*, mycoplasma hominis)	34	19.5
Trichomonas vaginalis	15	12.3
Chlamydia trachomatis	10	1.5
Cytomegalovirus	8	0
Neisseria gonorrhoeae	6	4.2
Herpes simplex virus	2	0
Treponema pallidum	1	0
Human immunodeficiency virus (HIV) type 1	1	0

*The incidence of new disease, at the follow-up examination: $n = 109$. Those found to be infected at the first visit or who were treated prophylactically were excluded (Jenny and others, 1990).

Table 3-2 *Sexually Transmitted Diseases in Sexually Assaulted Patients*

ETIOLOGY*	PREVALENCE†	SYMPTOMS	DIAGNOSIS‡	PRESCRIPTION§
Trichomoniasis (*trichomonas vaginalis*—protozoa)	12% in sexual assault patients without preexisting infection; no transmission by fomites	**F:** Asymptomatic or yellow-green malodorous vaginal discharge; vulvular irritation **M:** Urethritis or asymptomatic; does not colonize in mouth or gastrointestinal tract	Wet mount; culture; pap test may detect, but can be false positive	Metronidazole (Flagyl) 500mg by mouth twice daily for 7 days or 2 gm by mouth for single dose
Chlamydia (*chlamydia trachomatis*—intracellular, bacterial parasite)	2% in sexual assault patients without preexisting infection; highest among adolescents; incubation is greater than 10 days	**F:** Asymptomatic or vaginal discharge (mucoid-to-purulent), dysuria, pelvic pain **M:** Urethritis, dysuria, frequency, mucoid-to-purulent discharge	Culture from any site of penetration‖; Storage of specimen at 4°C (39°F) > 1 day, loss of viability	Doxycycline (Doxy 100) 100 mg by mouth twice daily for 7 days or azithromycin (Zithromax) 1 gm by mouth for single dose; for ages 15 and younger, use doxycycline; for pregnant women, use erythromycin base 500 mg by mouth four times daily for 7 days
Gonnorrhea (*neisseria gonorrhoeae*—gramnegative diplococcus)	4% in sexual assault patients without preexisting infection, highest in 15-to-19 year olds; coinfect with chlamydia is common; 3-to-21-day incubation	**F:** Asymptomatic or vaginal discharge; cystitis to pelvic inflammatory disease (PID) **M:** Dysuria, frequency, urethral discharge; conjunctiva, rectum, pharynx, and secondary sites	Culture from any site of penetration‖; organism viable 2 hours in water	Ceftriaxone (Rocephin) 125 mg or 250 mg intramuscular (IM) for single dose plus prescription for chlamydia treatment

*Trichomoniasis, chlamydia, gonorrhea, and bacterial vaginosis are the most commonly diagnosed STDs in sexual assault patients, the infection may have antedated the assault.
†$n = 204$ women and postmenarchal girls (Jenny and others, 1990)
‡All adolescents in the United States can consent to confidential diagnosis and prescription of STDs without parental consent or knowledge.
§Recommended regimen postassault (CDC, 1993); single-dose regimen may be preferred if completing the 7-day treatment is problematic.
‖Indirect technique not sensitive or specific enough for sexual assault (Stewart, 1992).

Table 3-2 *Sexually Transmitted Diseases in Sexually Assaulted Patients—cont'd*				
ETIOLOGY*	PREVALENCE†	SYMPTOMS	DIAGNOSIS‡	PRESCRIPTION§
Bacteria vaginosis Anaerobic bacteria (e.g., bacteroides species, mobiluncus) *Gardnerella vaginalis,* mycoplasma hominis	19% in sexual assault patients without preexisting infection; common in adolescents and adults—a marker of sexual activity¶	F: Asymptomatic to white maladorous vaginal discharge: pH> 4.5	Positive clue cells Positive whiff test (a fishy odor of vaginal discharge before or after addition of 10% potassium hydroxide); postpubescent pH> 4.5	Metronidazole (Flagyl) 500 mg by mouth twice daily for 7 days or 2 gm by mouth for single dose

¶Stewart, 1992
F: Female; M: Male
Adapted from Centers for Disease Control and Prevention: Sexually transmitted disease treatment guidelines, *MMWR* 42, No RR-14, 1993, US Department of Health and Human Services.

Prevention [CDC], 1993). Since these occur among sexually active women, their presence postassault does not signify acquisition during the assault.

The risk of acquiring a sexually transmitted disease as a result of an assault varies with the type of assault. Penile penetration of the vagina (vaginal, anal, oral), especially with ejaculation has the highest risk of STD transmission. Anal and oral penile penetration have lower risks of transmission (Jenny and others, 1990). Other factors increasing the risk of STD transmission are multiple offenders, as well as the larger the size of the inoculum, the greater the infectivity of the organisms transmitted and susceptibility of the victim to infection (Glaser, Hammerschlag, McCormack, 1989).

The prevalence of STDs in perpetrators was thought to be high because of the number and variety of their victims. However, Slaughter and Crowley (1993) found only 7% of 170 suspected male perpetrators and sex offenders had STDs. Chlamydia was the most common. There

were no positive tests for human immunodeficiency virus (HIV), of the 58 who were tested, and no increase in prevalence of STDs among those with previous histories of incarceration for sexual assault.

Table 3-2 describes the cause, prevalence, symptoms, diagnosis and treatment for the STDs typically identified in sexual assault patients. Table 3-3 describes other common STDs. Figures 3-7 to 3-16 show some STDs.

Amebiasis, shigellosis, giardia, Hepatitis A and B, and HIV are more prevalent in the homosexual community. Men, especially homosexual men who have been sexually assaulted, may need to be evaluated for these STDs (Glaser, Hammerschlag, McCormick, 1989).

HIV antibody seroconversion has been reported among persons whose only risk factor was sexual assault (CDC, 1993). The risk of acquiring HIV from sexual assault involving anal or vaginal penetration and exposure to ejaculate from a perpetrator with HIV is conservatively estimated to be at a minimum of two per 1000

Table 3-3	*More Sexually Transmitted Diseases in Sexually Assaulted Patients*			
ETIOLOGY	PREVALENCE	SYMPTOMS	DIAGNOSIS	PRESCRIPTION
Genital warts (human papillovirus [HPV]) genital type 6, 11	Parallels gonorrhea; highest in 16-to-25 year olds; 1 to 2 million per year in the United States; 13% to 38% are adolescent; incubation period: 2 up to 20 months	Pain or not, friable, pink wartlike lesions on vulva, vagina, cervix, anus, urethra, and glans penis; resolve and reappear	Appearance; HPV DNA test*; biopsy and histology; acetic acid 3% to 5%; turns white if positive (but false positives occur)	Remove with cryotherapy; Podofilox (Condylox) daily for 3 days then 4 days off; use< 0.5 mL daily; repeat cycle four times *Contraindications:* pregnancy
Genital herpes (Herpes simplex virus [HSV] Type II is the cause for 90% of genital herpes cases	30 million in the United States per year; 3 to 7 days incubation; transmission without recognized lesions[†]	Initial onset is asymptomatic to pruritis with papules—vesicles that ulcerate—on the vulva, vagina, and cervix, or the penile shaft, prepuce, or glans penis; some have recurring symptoms	Culture, cytology, serology, molecular techniques	Acyclovir (Zovirax) 200 mg by mouth five times daily for 7 to 10 days or until resolution; avoid chronic prescription and the development of drug-resistant strains; lesions recur
Hepatitis B (a virus of deoxyribonucleic [DNA] acid)	200,000 to 300,000 new cases per year in United States; high risk in multiple sex partners of HBV carriers, intravenous (IV) drug users, and homosexuals	Vague abdominal pain, anorexia, nausea, jaundice, arthralgia; also asymptomatic hepatitis	Test using HBsAg 1 to 2 months after exposure. Previous infection can be detected with anti-HBc, immunity can be demonstrated with anti-HBs, and the carrier state can be detected by HBsAg	Hepatitis immune globulin (HBIG) within 14 days after exposure 0.06 mL/kg for single dose; and Hepatitis B vaccine for prevention 1 mL IM deltoid at time of examination, 1, and 6 months

*Differentiate from verruca vulgaris, condylomata (secondary syphilis), epithelial papillae, sebaceous glands, molluscum, and contagiosum
[†]Stewart, 1992

Table 3-3 *More Sexually Transmitted Diseases in Sexually Assaulted Patients—cont'd*				
ETIOLOGY	PREVALENCE	SYMPTOMS	DIAGNOSIS	PRESCRIPTION
Syphilis (*treponema palidum*—anaerobic spirochete)	136,000 cases in United States annually; increasing in homosexual men and heterosexual women; 10-to-90-day incubation	*Phase 1:* Painless sore at site *Phase 2:* Skin rash *Phase 3:* Heart, nervous system involvement	VDRL, RPR, FTA-ABS Dark field examination of ulcer exudate	Benzathine penicillin G 2.4 million units IM; if allergy, doxycycline (Doxy 100) 100 mg by mouth twice daily for 14 days
Human immunodeficiency virus (HIV)	Risk with single heterosexual intercourse is less than 1%; risk with homosexuals is 2%; in 3 to 10 years between infection with HIV and acquired immunodeficiency syndrome (AIDS)	Varies from no illness to AIDS	3 and 6 months postassault HIV-1 antibody test, compared with initial results; also test perpetrator at suspect examination	Prophylactic treatment is not known to be effective

VDRL: venereal disease research laboratory
RPR: rapid plasmin reagin
FTA-ABS: fluorescent treponemal
Adapted from Centers for Disease Control and Prevention: Sexually transmitted disease treatment guidelines, *MMWR* 42, No RR-14, 1993, US Department of Health and Human Services.

contacts. The actual per-contact risk is higher if other factors are present, such as the presence of tissue injury, blood exposure, or the presence of inflammatory or ulcerative STDs (Gostin and others, 1994).

Consideration should be given to testing at 3 and 6 months after the assault because the majority of individuals with HIV have detectable antibodies within 3 to 6 months. Comparing baseline testing at the time of the initial examination with the follow-up testing is necessary to demonstrate that the assault resulted in HIV seroconversion, if other risks can be ruled out as causing the seroconversion. Tests that detect viral antigens rather than antibodies shorten the period from exposure to when HIV infection may be detected (Gostin and others, 1994). Testing is indicated especially when the perpetrator is a known intravenous (IV) drug user, has a sex partner who is a known IV drug user, has multiple sex partners, is homosexual, or is unknown (CDC, 1993). Testing also may help patients from the burden of wondering if they have contracted HIV. Testing enables patients to make informed decisions regarding their health, sexual or needle-sharing behavior, reproduction, breastfeeding, and parenting. Some states mandate preconviction testing. Federal law requires HIV testing for those convicted of rape (Gostin and others). Prophylactic

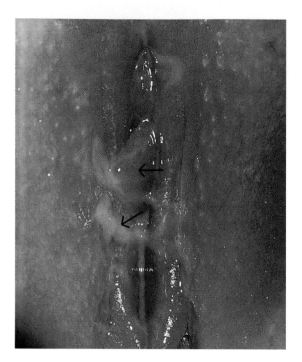

FIGURE 3-7 Gonorrhea (×15). Purulent vaginal discharge and vulvular redness is present in this preadolescent with a positive culture for *N. gonorrhoeae.*

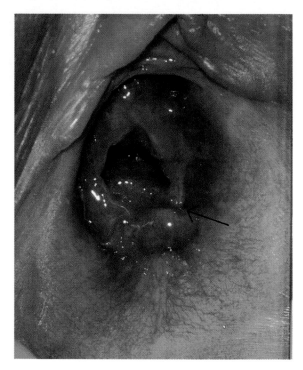

FIGURE 3-8 Chlamydia (×15). Reddened hymen and fossa navicularis with clear vaginal discharge is present in this Caucasian child with a positive *C. trachomatis* culture. There is a transection of the hymen at 3 o'clock.

treatment for HIV is not known to be effective and is generally not recommended (CDC, 1993).

If a protocol includes cultures, then a wet mount and culture of vaginal swabs should be obtained for *T. vaginalis,* bacterial vaginosis, and yeast. Cultures should be collected for *C. trachomatis* and *N. gonorrhoeae* from any site of penetration or attempted penetration. A serum sample should be obtained for syphilis and HIV, to compare with the 12-week specimen, if it is positive.

Prophylactic treatment for these infections (see Figures 3-8 and 3-9) is recommended by the CDC and is best started at the time of the initial medical-legal examination (CDC, 1993). Treatment is started at the time of the examination since only half may return for follow-up examinations, and 26% of those returning comply with the follow-up testing (Jenny and others, 1990) such as cultures. Single-dose alternatives are available for patients that may have difficulty following a 7-day regimen. Patients should be reminded that even with a single-dose regimen, a condom should be used until the end of the medication regimen.

OTHER NONASSAULT VARIATIONS

See Figures 3-17 to 3-22.

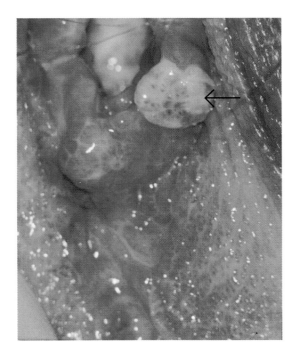

FIGURE 3-9 Genital warts, human papillovirus (HPV) (×15). Genital warts turn white when 3% acetic acid is applied.

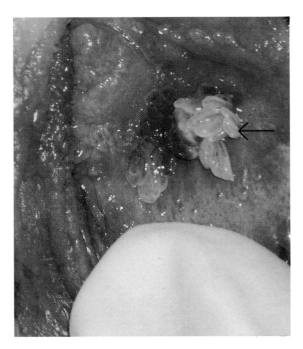

FIGURE 3-10 Genital warts (×15).

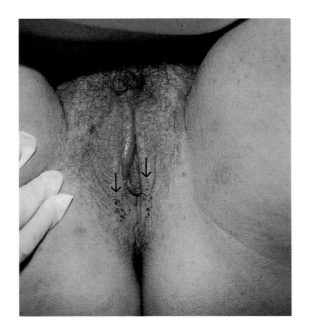

FIGURE 3-11 Genital herpes (35 mm) (Figures 3-11 to 3-14). Figures 3-11 through 3-14 are of the same patient. Herpetic ulcers with Toluidine Blue dye up-take are present. The labia are red and swollen and she complains of pain.

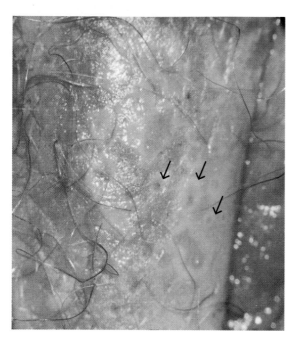

FIGURE 3-12 Herpetic ulcers without dye (×15). Ulcers are present that are not identified with arrows.

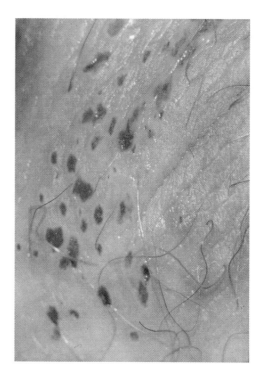

FIGURE 3-13 Herpetic ulcers with dye (×15).

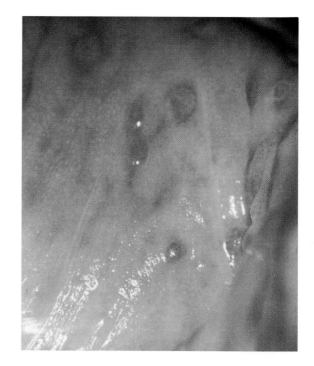

FIGURE 3-14 Herpetic lesions on the cervix (×15).

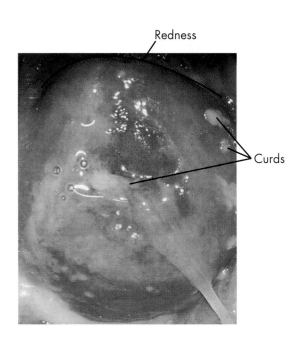

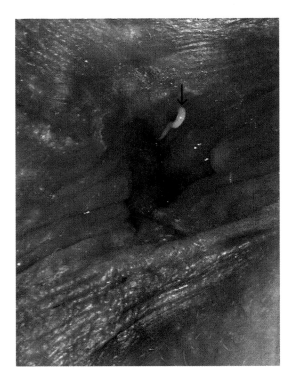

FIGURE 3-15 Candida on cervix (×15). Note the redness from 10 o'clock to 2 o'clock and the white curds.

FIGURE 3-16 A pinworm (×15).

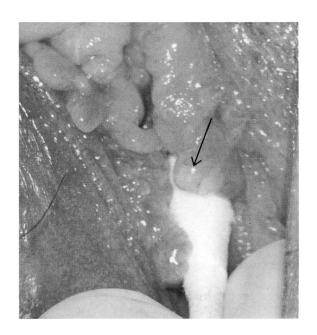

FIGURE 3-17 Hymenal cyst (×15). This patient was examined 20 hours postpenile vaginal penetration. Later, this sexually active, white 22-year-old admitted that the reported assault was consensual and she was angry with her boyfriend.

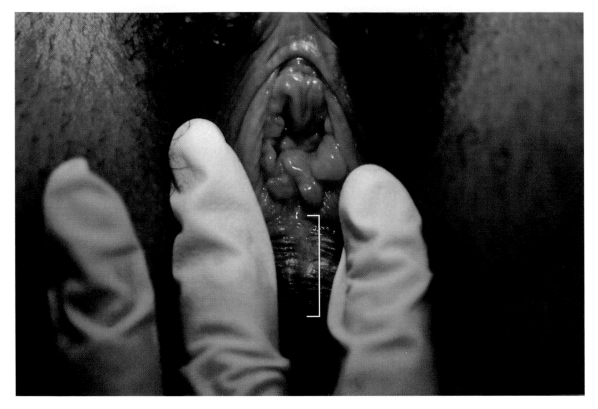

FIGURE 3-18   A 7-month-old episiotomy scar (35mm).

FIGURE 3-19   Urethral prolapse (×15). The patient was positioned in knee-chest for this photograph. This was diagnosed in the operating room after initial examination for complaints of blood on the patient's underwear. The history was negative for sexual abuse in this prepubescent female. She was discharged on antibiotics with gynecological follow-up.

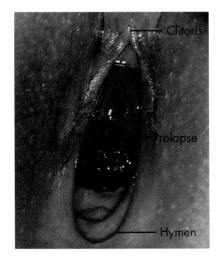

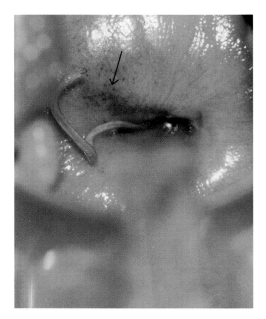

FIGURE 3-20 Cervical petechiae from 10 o'clock to 11 o'clock as a result of the string on an intrauterine device (×15).

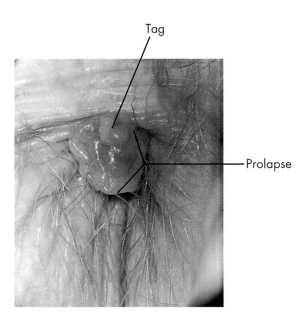

FIGURE 3-21 Anal tag on top of a prolapse (×15).

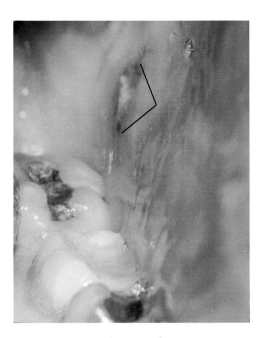

FIGURE 3-22 Buccal mucosa bite injury (×15). Injury was self-inflicted, 6 hours old.

REFERENCES

Bays J and others: Changes in hymenal anatomy during examination of prepubertal girls for possible sexual abuse, *Adolesc Pediatr Gyn* 3:42, 1990.

Berenson AB: Conditions that may be misdiagnosed as sexual abuse. In *Mimic Abuse* [Online], 1996.

Centers for Disease Control and Prevention: Sexually transmitted disease treatment guidelines, *MMWR* 42, No RR-14, 1993, US Department of Health and Human Services (new guidelines expected in 1997).

Danielson RW: Vaginal ulcers caused by tampons, *Am J Ob Gyn* 146:547, 1983.

Dudgeon D, Paidas CW: Trauma to the vulva and vagina. In Carpenter SE, Rock JA, editors: *Pediatric and adolescent gynecology,* New York, 1992, Raven.

Emans SJ and others: Hymenal findings in adolescent women: impact of tampon use and consensual sexual activity, *J Pediatr* 125:153, 1994.

Friedrich EG, Siegesmund KA: Tampon associated vaginal ulcerations, *Ob Gyn* 55:149, 1980.

Gibbons M, Vincent EC: Childhood sexual abuse, *Am Fam Phys* 49:1, 1994.

Glaser JB, Hammerschlag MR, McCormack WM: Epidemiology of sexual transmitted diseases in rape victims, *Rev Infect Dis* 11:246, 1989.

Glaser JB, Hammerschlag MR, McCormack WM: Sexually transmitted diseases in victims of sexual assault, *N Engl J Med* 315:625, 1986.

Gostin LO and others: HIV testing, counseling and prophylaxis after sexual assault, *J Am Med Assn* 271:1436, 1994.

Gray MJ, Norton P, Treadwell, K: Tampon-induced injuries, *Ob Gyn* 58:667, 1981.

Heger A: Personal communication, November, 1996.

Jenny C and others: Sexually transmitted diseases in victims of rape, *N Engl J Med* 322:713, 1990.

Lauber AA, Souma, ML: Use of Toluidine Blue for documentation of traumatic intercourse, *Ob Gyn* 60:644, 1982.

Murphy SM: Rape, sexually transmitted diseases and human immunodeficiency virus infection, *Internat J STD AIDS* 1:79, 1990.

Slaughter L, Crowley, S: *Prevalence of sexually transmitted diseases in sex offenders.* Paper presented at the North American Association of Pediatric and Adolescent Gynecology, April 1993.

Stewart D: Sexually transmitted diseases. In Heger A, Emans SJ, editors: *Evaluation of the sexually abused child,* New York, 1992, Oxford University Press.

SUGGESTED READINGS

Baker RB: Anal fissure produced by examination for sexual abuse, *Am J Dis Child* 145:848, 1991.

Beebe D K: Emergency management of the adult female rape victim, *Am Fam Phy* 43:2041, 1991.

Forster GE and others: Incidence of sexually transmitted diseases in rape victims during 1984, *Genitourinary Med* 62:267, 1986.

4 CARE OF THE SEXUALLY ASSAULTED PATIENT

A systematic approach to the care of the sexually assaulted patient helps to ensure that the highest quality evidence is collected while initial emotional care is provided and teaching is planned. *Care, collect, conclude,* and *continue* are the goals of the examiner (Table 4-1).

Emotional *care* for sexually assaulted adolescents and adults with rape trauma syndrome may be provided during the medical-legal examination by using techniques of critical incident stress debriefing (CISD) (Mitchell, 1996).

The medical-legal examination provides for evidence *collection. Concluding* the examination consists of teaching, offering treatment with medication, connecting to resources, and checking the evidence and the documents used to record the medical-legal examination. The examiner *continues* with the follow-up examination to evaluate healing to reinforce teaching and refer for further care.

EMOTIONAL CARE

Rape trauma syndrome (RTS) and posttraumatic stress disorder (PTSD) are two emotional states that may follow sexual assault (Burgess, Fehder, Hartman, 1995; Ochberg, 1988). An understanding of these states and approaches like critical incident stress debriefing (CISD), (Mitchell, 1996) helps to ensure the patient receives compassionate care during the medical-legal examination and helps to initiate the emotional recovery process. Stabilization of the patient's emotional equilibrium is one goal of the specialized sexual assault examiners (Lynch, 1993). After the examination, patients are referred for essential postassault counseling, which attempts to redirect them into therapeutic coping patterns rather than defensive ones

Table 4-1	*Care Components*	
PROCESS	TECHNIQUE	PARTS
Emotional *care*	Critical incident stress debriefing (CISD)	Introduce Explore Inform
Collect evidence	Medical-legal examination	Prepare Interview Examine
Conclude	Concluding the initial examination	Teach Treat Connect Check
Continue	Follow-up examination	Examine Teach Refer

and to reestablish a sense of control (Burgess and others, 1995).

Emotional care has indirect effects as well. The manner in which the examination is conducted influences the quality of the history, the cooperation during the examination, and the patient's attitude toward taking legal measures. Perceiving an attitude of acceptance by the examiner facilitates the patient's emotional recovery (Minden, 1989). Conversely, the judgmental and impersonal manner by which some patients perceive care has caused them to withdraw their testimony (Schwartz, Clear, 1980).

Rape Trauma Syndrome

A pattern of moderate-to-severe symptoms of rape trauma syndrome (RTS) occurs in most victims of sexual assault (Burgess and others, 1995). The minority of patients report mild symptoms or none at all (Burgess and others, 1995). If severe symptoms last longer than 1 month, posttraumatic stress disorder (PTSD) may be present.

RTS and the forms of PTSD are as follows:

RTS: Symptoms less than 1 month

PTSD Acute: Symptoms less than 3 months

PTSD Chronic: Symptoms 3 months or more

PTSD Delayed: Symptoms begin after 6 months (American Psychiatric Association [APA], 1994).

RTS is a cluster of varying degrees of biopsychosocial and behavioral responses to the profound fear of death that patients experience during the assault. Self-preservation is the aim of the symptoms. All the symptoms are valid because that is how the patient is responding to the assault. The ability to cope with the incident depends on the nature of the assault, other stressors, the patient's preexisting function, coping skills, and available support systems (Burgess and others, 1995; Oakleaf, 1995). Techniques of CISD (Mitchell, Everly, 1996), may be used by the examiner to help initiate the recovery process. Patients are referred for essential postassault counseling.

RTS may be divided into the acute and the reorganization phases (Hartman, Burgess, 1988).

ACUTE PHASE

This phase may last a few days to a few weeks after the incident.

Emotional responses: Patients show a wide range of emotions that fit into the categories of expressed or controlled styles. Initially there is disbelief and shock. This allows for an emotional "time-out" to process the experience. If the assault was particularly brutal, the patient may block out the incident. There is major disruption in the patient's life.

Expressed style: There is anger, fear, anxiety, restlessness during the interview, crying and sobbing while describing specific acts of the perpetrator, as well as smiling when certain issues are stated.

Controlled style: The feelings of the patient are masked by a calm, composed, subdued affect. The patient may sit calmly, answer questions logically, and downplay any fear, anger, and anxiety.

Physical responses: Most typically, there is skeletal muscle tension, general soreness throughout, and specific areas of pain that were the targets of the assault. There may be gastrointestinal irritability, genitourinary disturbance, sleeping, eating, sexual disruption, and nightmares in which the assault experience is relived. These may result from the physical trauma or may be psychosomatic.

REORGANIZATION PHASE

Patients undergo a wide range of emotions and physical responses with the purpose of reorganizing their life after the assault. Many survivors feel a need to "get away." They may change their phone number, residence, job, and school. They may withdraw socially or want to be with other people constantly, depending on their personality and the situation of the assault. Increased motor activity, repeated and disturbing nightmares, development of fears and phobic reactions to the circumstances of the assault are apparent.

ADDITIONAL SYMPTOMS IN EITHER PHASE

Patients experience shame, self-blame, subjugation evidenced as powerlessness, morbid hatred of the perpetrator, vengefulness, paradoxical gratitude for the gift of life, feeling dirty, sexual inhibition, mistrust, resignation and despair, panic on seeing the scene of the assault or the perpetrator, feelings of revictimization through participation in various care systems, and socioeconomic status downward drift (Oakleaf, 1995; Ochberg, 1993).

Posttraumatic Stress Disorder

According to the *Diagnostic and Statistical Manual of Mental Disorders, Fourth Edition* (DSM-IV) (APA, 1994), PTSD occurs when certain behavioral criteria are evident in the patient (see Box 4-1).

Box 4-1	*Posttraumatic Stress Disorder*

A. Duration of the symptoms is *more than 1 month* and the symptoms were not present before the trauma. When RTS extends beyond 1 month, with the remaining characteristics (B through F), PTSD is present.

B. A person has been exposed to a *traumatic event* in which *both* of the following were present:

1. The person experienced, witnessed, or was confronted with an event that involved actual or threatened death or serious injury, or a threat to the physical integrity of self or others.

2. The person's response involved intense fear, helplessness, or horror

C. The traumatic event is *persistently reexperienced* in one or more of the following ways:

1. Involuntary intrusive thoughts
2. Recurrent distressing dreams of the event
3. Flashback episodes
4. Intense psychological distress at exposure to cues that resemble an aspect of the traumatic event.
5. Physiological distress on exposure to cues that resemble an aspect of the traumatic event

D. Three or more *avoidance symptoms:*

1. Avoids thoughts, feelings, or talk associated with the trauma
2. Avoids activities, places, or people that arouse recollections of the trauma
3. Inability to recall aspects of the trauma
4. Diminished interest or participation in significant activities
5. Feeling of detachment from others
6. Restricted range of affect (e.g., unable to have loving feelings)
7. Sense of a foreshortened future (e.g., does not expect to have a career, marriage, or a normal life span).

E. At least two symptoms of *increased arousal:*

1. Difficulty falling or staying asleep
2. Irritability or outbursts of anger
3. Difficulty concentrating
4. Hypervigilance
5. Exaggerated startle response

F. The disturbance causes *clinically significant distress* or impairment in social, occupational, or other important areas of functioning.

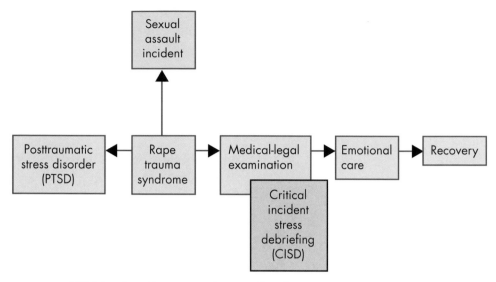

FIGURE 4-1   Posttraumatic stress disorder to recovery continuum.

Critical Incident Stress Debriefing

Critical incident stress debriefing (CISD) (Mitchell, Everly, 1996) techniques by the examiner help the patient control the postassault anxiety, decrease the intensity of the incident and begin to build self-worth and control. CISD helps resolve RTS and resist the movement toward PTSD disorder (Mitchell, 1996) (Figure 4-1). The techniques should be integrated throughout the medical-legal examination.

CISD consists of *introducing* the setting, *exploring* the incident and *informing* the patient. Deliberately using techniques of CISD during the history and examination launches the recovery process.

INTRODUCE THE SETTING

The examiner should connect with the patient through eye contact, tone, and body language.

- Ask patient's name and use name throughout the medical-legal examination.

- Introduce personnel and identify the setting.
- Ensure the patients that they will have privacy during the examination.
- Explain confidentiality, invite questions and request personal preferences; comply with them as possible. Confidentiality may not be maintained in child abuse cases when reporting is required by law.
- Offer options, and follow the decision that is chosen.
- Emphasize that giving consent for the examination is under the patient's control, as is his or her cooperation with the legal system to proceed in prosecuting the perpetrator.

EXPLORE THE INCIDENT

- Encourage a chronological report of the incident. "Tell me what happened, in order."
- Paraphrase for clarification: "What I hear you saying is. . ."
- Validate feelings: Her comments of, "I

couldn't do anything. I was at his mercy," can be responded with, "It sounds like you felt helpless. How did you feel? What is the worst thing about this event?"

- Accept silence, crying, and anger.
- Affirm that it takes courage to relate the details. Remind the patient that "restorying" repeatedly helps recovery.
- Refrain from expressing surprise or disgust.
- Ask, "Did anything like this ever happen before?" Those who have a previous history of victimization may have a more profound loss of self-esteem and may be more vulnerable and prone to emotional crisis. The potential for self-harm should be evaluated and then emergent emotional care should be obtained as needed.
- Ask more than once, "Is there anything else that might be important for me to know?"

INFORM THE PATIENT
- Remind them repeatedly, "It is not your fault. You are safe here," "You did what you could."
- Summarize the incident as understood by the examiner.
- Normalize emotions, "It's normal for you to feel powerless and violated."
- In response to a patient's stated intentions to harm the perpetrator, remind the patient that he or she would also be the perpetrator of a crime. The legal and judicial system works with victims to apprehend, bring to trial, and punish their perpetrators.
- Initiate an emergent referral if patient expresses the intention to harm themselves.
- Identify the power that patients have to control their recoveries, to express their needs without feeling guilt, to express anger without losing control, to try new

experiences and plan time to care for themselves.
- Clarify myths and reality related to sexual assault (see Appendix A).
- Provide written material identifying resources available (books, support groups, rape crisis centers) (see Appendix B).
- Review and explain support systems that are available. Encourage the patient to confide in a family member or friend for ongoing support. Explain to the primary support person that the patient will need to "restory" repeatedly. Direct the support person to avoid statements that would heighten self-blame, such as, "You asked for it," or, "Why did you go there?"
- Remind them that victim services will explain the local support systems, and in some locations is accessible by phone.
- An advocate should be available during all stages of the examination if approved by the patient. The advocate supports and comforts the victim during history and examination, helps with information, and contacts with community resources, and is available to accompany the patient during the trial. The advocate asks the patient, "May I call you in a few days?" also requesting phone number(s) at which the patient can be reached. If no advocate is available, the significant other may serve as the emotional support for the patient during the examination. Teach this support person exactly what is expected of them before beginning either the history or physical portion of the medical-legal examination.
- Encourage patient to contact a professional counselor (psychological counselor, social worker, and/or a spiritual counselor) experienced in caring for sexually assaulted pa-

tients. Referral names and numbers should be written as part of the follow-up care instructions (see Appendix C).

COLLECT EVIDENCE

The Medical-Legal Examination

The sexual assault history and examination begins with triage and immediate treatment of life-threatening injuries. A systematic approach to the care of the sexually assaulted patient helps to ensure that the highest quality objective evidence is collected by the examiner while initial emotional care and teaching is planned. A consistent technique helps ensure a complete examination and minimizes the potential for loss of evidence and cross-contamination between anatomical sites. It is admissible in court. It is more defensible in court during cross-examination to have conducted the medical-legal examination according to standard protocol.

It is the role of the examiner to remain unbiased, identify the injury or lack of injury, and determine if the findings demonstrate sexual contact and whether they are consistent with the history and timing of the reported event (Slaughter, Brown 1991). In maintaining an impartial perspective the examiner should understand that consensual intercourse can result in injury and nonconsensual intercourse can have no evidence of trauma (Lauber, Souma, 1982; Slaughter, 1997). Therefore the presence or absence of injury alone is not sufficient to conclude whether the reported intercourse was nonconsensual or not. The evidence collected in the medical-legal examination is only part of the evidence used to clarify the reported sexual assault.

The evidentiary examination yields the highest quality evidence if it is done within 72 hours from the time of the incident. Beyond 72 hours postassault, most trace evidence is lost and significant healing of genital and nongenital trauma has occurred. The examination then is no longer emergent but still necessary. Law enforcement may request an examination beyond 72 hours postassault, particularly a colposcopic examination if there is pain or bleeding. Evidence of healing injuries may be documented.

History and Physical Examination of the Adult Female

The steps in the medical-legal examination are (1) preparation, (2) history, and (3) physical examination. Appendix D lists highlights of the examination in a one-page format. The following detailed, exemplary protocol for the female patient is based on the California Office of Criminal Justice Planning (OCJP) requirements (see Appendix E, Form 923). Other local jurisdictions, states, and crime laboratories may have different requirements and forms (Young and others, 1992). The examiner must know the requirements in their jurisdiction and keep up with those changing requirements.

Prepare

1. Before the patient arrives, prepare and check the examination room and equipment. Once the examination is started, the examiner must remain in visual contact with the evidence to maintain the chain of custody. The following should be available during the examination:
   - Crime laboratory "assault kit" and extra swabs as indicated
   - Form for documenting the consents, history, physical examination, and evidence, such as the Form 923, Office of Criminal Justice Planning (OCJP). Appendix E provides an example of Form 923.

- Identification labels for evidence according to Association for Standards of Test Materials (ASTM) standards (ASTM, 1992) should include the patient's name, date of birth, medical record number, time, date, contents, location where taken, institutional site, and examiner's name.
- 35 mm camera with macro lens and photo or slide film, colposcope, microscope, Wood's lamp or alternative light source with appropriate yellow lens filter, and swab dryer. Video colposcopy with digital printer if available.
- Clothing and hygiene kit for the patient after the examination
- Medications according to the latest CDC recommendations
- Written referral and follow-up care recommendations

2. Explain examination procedures to the patient and obtain the following informed *consents* for physical examination: evidence collection, HIV testing, photography, transmission of information and evidence to law enforcement, and prophylactic treatment of pregnancy.
   - An advocate should attend to the patient throughout the history and the physical examination. The advocate may want to contact the patient later and attend court with her or him.

3. Before proceeding with the history, collect oral evidence and blood specimens. Oral swabs and slides are collected if it is within 6 hours of the assault and there is a history of oral copulation. Secretor status is always collected. Then refreshments and oral care can be offered without interfering with evidence. Drawing blood specimens and collecting urine for medications will prevent the effect of time on toxicology levels.
   - *Slides:* Prepare two dry-mount slides for presence of sperm from swabs of the lower buccal mucosa. Dry, label, and document.
   - *STD cultures:* If indicated, take culture of oropharynx for gonorrhea and chlamydia. Agencies treat for potential STDs without culturing. Dry, label, and document.
   - *Secretor status:* Have patient thoroughly moisten half of a sterile gauze pad or paper wafer with saliva. Handle the specimen with tweezers or gloves to avoid contaminating the specimen with secretions from the examiner, or ask the patient to handle it. This specimen is used to determine if the patient secretes their ABO blood type into body fluids. Dry, label, and document.

Draw the following blood specimens (tube type may vary with laboratory):
   - ABO and serology (purple)
   - Blood alcohol (gray) if within 24 hours of the assault
   - Syphilis (rapid plasma reagin [RPR], hepatitis B (HBV), HIV, human chorionic gonadotropin (HCG); HCG levels may be obtained by urine or blood testing. HCG will appear in the blood or urine of pregnant women as early as 10 days after conception.

4. If the patient must void immediately, collect the urine in two specimens, one for toxicology and one for pregnancy and the presence of spermatozoa. The tissue wipe should be dried, labeled, and submitted with the other evidence. These urine specimens would have otherwise been collected after the Wood's lamp evaluation as listed in Visual Examination of the Body Surface, pp. 95-97.

Interview

1. Record the detailed history of sexual assault on a standard examination form, such as the Form 923 (see Appendix E). The history and the examination are integral components of the medical-legal examination. The history is critical in guiding the subsequent examination for forensic evidence. For example, if the patient states that she was bitten on her back, the examiner should examine and plan to photograph the patient's back. The history is also corroborated by physical findings. The history is best taken from the patient using open-ended questions that encourage the patient to relate the details. Avoid questions that allow for simple yes-or-no answers. Record the patient's own words using quotation marks.

The history may seem fragmented yet may be as accurate as the patient is capable. Fragmented recollection occurs because a threat to life floods the noradrenergic system and triggers the opioid system (Burgess, Hartman, 1995), causing an interruption in memory pathways. The examiner may need to piece the history together, then verify the accuracy of the recording with the patient.

Most settings have a translator for non–English-speaking patients, or a certified translator for many languages is available 24 hours per day for a fee.* Developmental and culturally appropriate communications improve the accuracy and comfort of the history. For example, medical terminology (clarified) may be more acceptable to the elderly than would street language.

*Services available through the AT&T Language Line at 1-800-528-5888.

The following should be included in the history:

- Date and time of the assault
- Perpetrator characteristics: age, gender, race, relationship to patient, height, weight, sexual dysfunction
- Manner of the assault: number of assailants, the exact threats, and/or weapons and restraints
- Location of the assault: address, appearance of the surroundings (i.e., bed, floor, table where assault occurred)
- Position of patient during the assault
- Patient's own words describing the assault, in quotes "I hit my leg on the wood box when he pushed me onto the bed."
- Sequence of contact and penetration:
  -Vaginal contact: with what, duration of contact, and the number of times. Was there orgasm by perpetrator or patient? Was foam, jelly, condom, or other lubrication used?
  -Anal contact: with what and number of times
  -Oral copulation of genitals or anus: By the patient or perpetrator? Manual stimulation? By patient or perpetrator?
  -Ejaculation: If yes, describe where. Condom used? Fondling, licking, sucking, or kissing? Describe.
- Actions following the assault: Douche (when, with what), bath, shower, defecate, urinate, brush teeth or gargle, remove or inserted tampon, change clothing, change underwear, ate, drank
- Injury to the perpetrator: "I scratched his head really hard." Fingernail scrapings of epithelial cells matched with photographs of scratch marks (Figure 4-2) may corroborate the history.

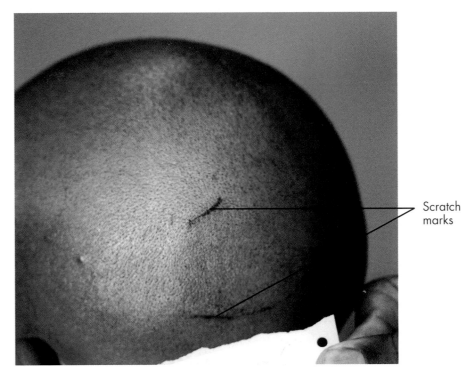

Scratch marks

FIGURE 4-2   Scratch marks on the back of the head (35mm).

2. Physical and emotional symptoms
3. Pertinent past medical history, including last menstrual period, prior sexual experience, parity and medication use such as estrogen. If patient has had consensual intercourse within the last 72 hours, identify the partner.
4. Additional information: Alcohol or drug use by patient or perpetrator, unknown drugs given by the perpetrator to the patient, prior surgeries, or other treatment that may affect the evidence. Knowledge of prior history of victimization can help the examiner be prepared for differentiating previous findings from acute findings.

Examine

This section includes principles to follow for the examination and a detailed explanation of the physical examination of the female patient. Highlights of the examination are included in Appendix D.

Universal precautions should be followed. Gloves should be latex, powder-free to avoid powder dust on the camera.

Principles. The principles of "control, dry, package, label, and document" should be followed in processing all specimens.

Control Swabs. A control swab is taken of an area that is unaffected and adjacent to the actual swab site. If the history reveals oral contact with

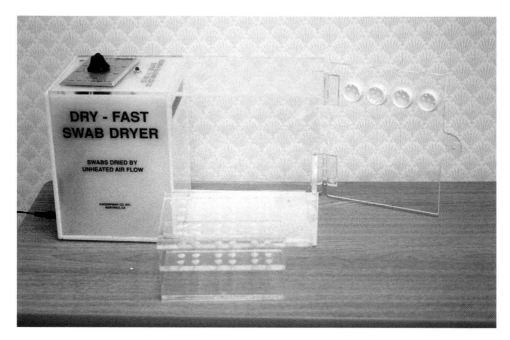

FIGURE 4-3   Swab dryer.

the left breast, the right breast would be swabbed with a sterile water swab as a control. Roll swabs over the skin. Do not rub. Use sterile water to moisten swabs. Avoid saline, which crystallizes, and tap water, which may contain DNA contaminants.

Dry. All specimens should be cool-air dried (60 minutes) in a swab dryer (Figure 4-3) before packaging to avoid overgrowth of contaminants and deterioration of the evidence. Wet mounts should be evaluated under the microscope for spermatozoa and organisms, then dried before packaging.

Package. All evidence should be inserted into the appropriate paper envelope or other container after it is dry at the end of the examination. Trace evidence should be placed on a self-sticking note and bindled (Figure 4-4) to prevent loss. The self-sticking note secures evidence as small as a single fiber. The bindle keeps

each piece of trace evidence separate. It should then be enclosed in a larger evidence envelope. Do *not* use plastic bags, which cause evidence to deteriorate.

Label. All the bags, envelopes, bindles, slide containers, and clothing containers should be labeled with the patient's name, date of birth, medical record number, time, date, contents, location where taken, institutional site, and examiner's name. At the end of the examination, the envelopes and other evidence containers are placed in a larger bag. Each item of clothing should be placed in a separate paper bag. Clothing is bagged separately from examination evidence. The large bag is closed, sealed with a sticker, dated, and initialed by the examiner. Labeling is performed the same way for all evidence.

Document. On examination form, describe and locate all injuries on a diagram on the ex-

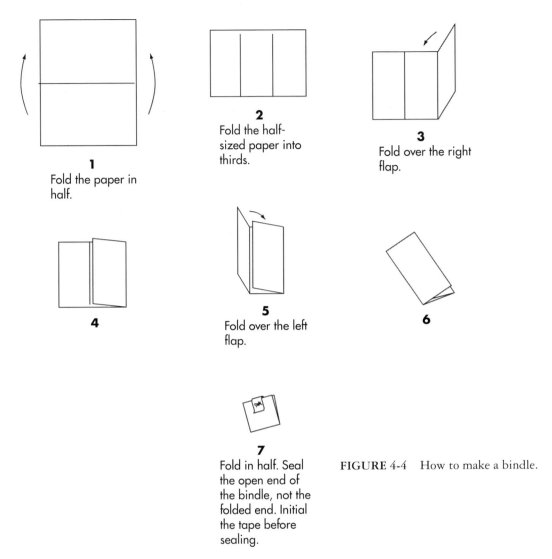

1
Fold the paper in half.

2
Fold the half-sized paper into thirds.

3
Fold over the right flap.

4

5
Fold over the left flap.

6

7
Fold in half. Seal the open end of the bindle, not the folded end. Initial the tape before sealing.

FIGURE 4-4   How to make a bindle.

amination form. Includes size, depth, and shape of the injury, as well as the distance from landmarks to the injury. Note whether the injury was visualized without magnification. Record findings from each anatomical site including those sites identified in the history. For example, if there is a history of a bite, identify the exact location and describe it, even if the area appears normal because the bruise may have not yet developed. Document tenderness on palpation. Identify Toluidine Blue dye uptake. List each specimen obtained including control specimens and from what site the specimens were obtained. If law enforcement defers the collection of a specimen, record this with name, badge number, date and time. Summarize significant findings, if physical findings support the history and whether there is evidence of sexual contact (Slaughter, Brown, 1991). Document by photographing (35mm and magnified) to support written findings. See Photodocumentation, pp. 119-120).

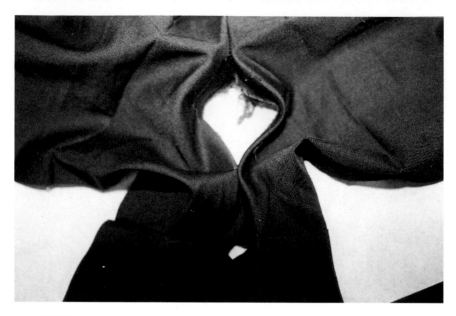

FIGURE 4-5 Torn shorts at the crotch and anterior to the crotch.

Details of the history and physical examination

Note Appearance. Note general condition and affect of the patient. Key words may be calm, shaking, crying, wringing hands, maintains eye contact, follows directions. The appearance of the clothing if worn during the assault are recorded. Take 35mm photos of the patient dressed. Take pictures of torn sections of clothing worn during the assault (Figure 4-5) and stains, with and without a photomacrographic scale (Figure 4-6)

Collect Clothing. If patient is still wearing the clothes she wore during the assault, scan clothing with the Wood's lamp (Figure 4-7) in a darkened room to identify stains that fluoresce. If there is a wet stain on the clothes, allow the wet areas to dry before putting garments into a bag. Do not swab. Label and document.

Have patient disrobe while standing on two layers of white paper on the floor (Figure 4-8).

The bottom paper helps keep the top sheet of paper clean. Provide the patient a gown and blanket. Collect under and outer clothing that was worn during or immediately after the assault. Do not shake the clothing nor disrupt a tear in the clothing. If the patient has showered and has changed her clothing, collect the underpants. Tell law enforcement if worn, unwashed clothing or linens used during or after the assault are accessible elsewhere. Fold each garment to prevent stains or foreign materials from being lost. Avoid folding a stain. Put each item in a separate paper bag. Paper bags allow secretions to dry and prevent bacterial deterioration of the specimen.

If foreign objects are identified on the clothing, first take photographs, then place each foreign object in separate envelopes. Label and document. Record the description of each item of clothing taken. Collect the top sheet of paper on which the patient has been disrobing, as any trace evidence may have fallen out onto the

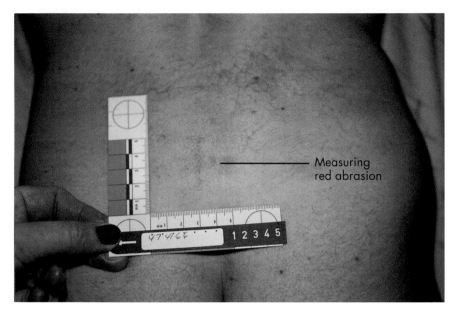

FIGURE 4-6 Photomacrographic scale (35mm). (*From American Board of Forensic Odontologists: Guidelines for bite mark analysis*, J Am Dent Assn *122:383, 1986;* NOTE: The photomacrographic scale is available from Lighting Powder Co., Inc., 1230 Hoyt St. S.E., Salem, OR 97302-2121, (503)585-9900, (800)852-0300.)

paper. Fold the top sheet into a bindle (see Figure 4-4) to secure trace evidence within. Label and document.

If clothing is wet, lay each item on a sheet of clean, unused paper and allow to dry. Gently fold each article of clothing and place in a paper bag. Label and document.

Visual Examination of the Body Surface.
Conduct a head-to-toe visual examination of the body. Use a standard technique, from top to bottom and outside to inside. A clock face is useful to locate sites of injury. TEARS is a helpful acronym in describing findings (Slaughter, Brown, 1991):

T   Tears or lacerations and/or tenderness
E   Ecchymosis
A   Abrasions
R   Redness
S   Swelling

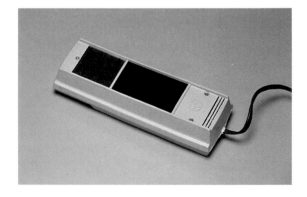

FIGURE 4-7 Wood's lamp (35mm). (*From Seidel HM et al:* Mosby's guide to physical examination, *ed 3, St Louis, 1995, Mosby.*)

Describe and locate by measuring any TEARS, adherent foreign matter, birthmarks, tattoos, burns, scars, or lesions. Be alert for bruising, lacerations, or blood or debris behind the ears, in front and back of neck, and in the

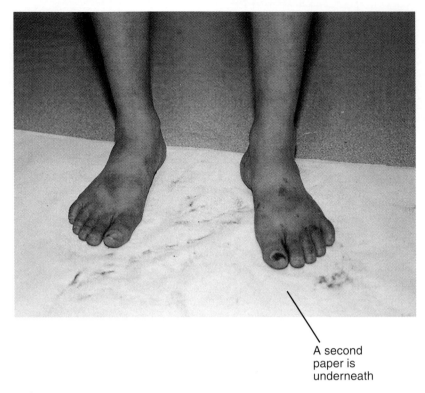

A second
paper is
underneath

FIGURE 4-8 Two sheets of paper used while disrobing to collect clothing evidence. Trace evidence may also be identified while disrobing.

scalp. Photograph, with and without a photomacrographic scale (Hyzer, Krauss, 1988). In photographing, proceed using the principles of wide-to-narrow focus and decreasing-to-increasing magnification. Consider using colposcopic magnification. (See Colposcopy and Photodocumentation, pp. 119-120). After photographing, trace evidence may be collected with tweezers or swab, or it may be scraped and placed onto the adhesive of a self-sticking note, then bindled to avoid loss. Trace evidence (grass, dirt, sand fibers, and sticks [Figure 4-9]) can be critical in verifying history, locating a crime site, identifying a suspect, or linking a victim and suspect. Package, label, and document.

With a Wood's lamp or alternative light source, scan the entire body, including the perineum, before allowing the patient to urinate (see Wood's Lamp and Alternative Light Source, p. 122). Swabs are obtained from areas on the body that fluoresce scratches, bitemarks, semen, and stains. For moist secretions, use a dry swab. For dry secretions, use a swab moistened with sterile water. Avoid scraping semen to collect it, because it may disintegrate. Take a control specimen on an adjacent area of skin not contaminated by secretions. The swabs are dried in cool air using a swab dryer and labeled "Wood's lamp finding" or "alternative light finding," along with the location on the body where it was collected. Document.

For a positive Wood's lamp finding in the pubic hair, clip the entire area that fluoresces. Dry, package, label, and document.

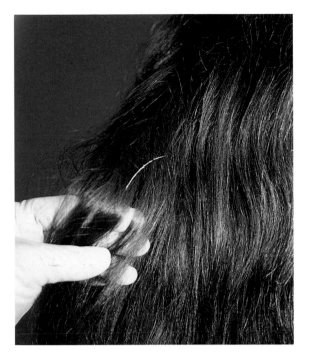

FIGURE 4-9   Trace evidence: a stick in the hair.

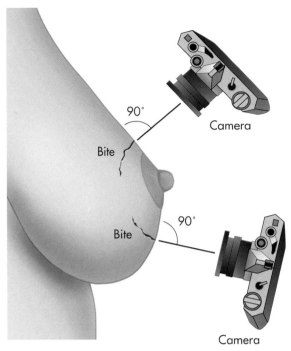

FIGURE 4-10   Photographing a curved surface while maintaining a 90-degree angle.

Collect two urine specimens, one for toxicology and one for pregnancy evaluation and presence of spermatozoa. Patient should avoid wiping to prevent evidence loss. However, used tissues are included as evidence. Dry tissues, label, and document.

Bite Marks. Take photographs with and without the photomacrographic scale. The entire bite mark should be recorded in one photographic frame. If the bite mark is on a curved surface as on the breast, the photograph should be taken in two steps. One photograph at 90 degrees from the upper dental arch marks and one photograph at 90 degrees from the lower dental arch marks (Rawson and others, 1986) (Figure 4-10). Colposcopic photographs of bite marks help to evaluate the depth and the fea-

tures of the teeth (Golden, 1996) Evaluate bite marks again at the end of the examination. Repeat photographs then, if more distinct features have developed.

Bite Mark Swab. Roll a moistened swab along the inside dental arch marks for saliva residue. Repeat the same procedure for the center of the bite mark and then slightly below the bite marks. Obtain a total of three swab specimens. Use another swab to take a control on an area not bitten.

If the patient reports other sites of oral contact, swab those areas and obtain a control. Dry, label, and document. These swabs are obtained to determine secretor status of the perpetrator. Of the U.S. population, 80% are secretors who reveal their blood type (A, B, O, AB) in all body fluids—saliva, seminal fluid, tears, or perspiration. This information can help rule out suspects. For example, if a suspect is a B secretor, and type A was demonstrated on the swabs of a type O patient, the discrepancy can be demonstrated.

Bite Mark Castings. If the marks have broken the skin or left an indentation, promptly have an examiner trained in casting techniques or the forensic odontologist evaluate for the possibility of taking a casting of the indentation. See Castings of Bite Marks on pp. 116-119.

Head Examination and Specimen Collection. Place a small paper sheet under the patient's head, comb the hair on the head to collect all debris and foreign hairs. Place the comb, along with the strands of hair, and collected debris on the sheet. Bindle the sheet, place it in an envelope. Label and document.

Cut 12 to 20 exemplar hairs from various areas of the head. These hairs should be cut close to the scalp or pulled as required by the local crime laboratory. If the crime laboratory requires pulled hairs, they are most easily pulled if the examiner or patient makes the skin tight and pulls a few hairs close to the skin, at a time. These hair standards are used to rule out the patient as the source of evidence hairs found on the clothing or the body. The examiner should maintain communications with the crime lab to stay updated on revised local requirements. Bindle the hairs, package, label, and document.

Fingernails. Take photographs of hands extended outward on blue background. Photograph freshly broken nails (Figure 4-11). Clip off any broken parts of the nail, preserving the broken edge. Place the nail on the sticky side of

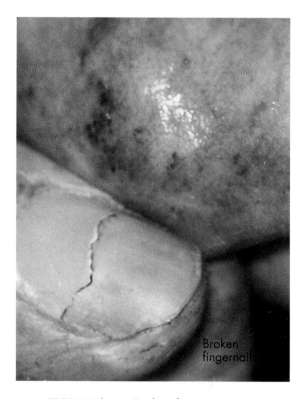

FIGURE 4-11   Broken fingernail (×15).

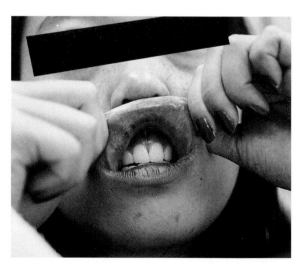

FIGURE 4-12   Upper lip eversion performed by the patient (35mm).

a self-sticking note. Use toothpicks to scrape under the fingernails. Place the scrapings from under the fingernails of each hand on the sticky part of separate self-sticking notes. Bindle with the toothpicks and scissors used to collect the evidence and insert bindles into an envelope. Label and document.

The Lips and Mouth. Examine for TEARS on the outside and opposing surfaces of upper and lower lips, mucosal surfaces of lips and upper and lower frenula by having the patient evert the lips (Figure 4-12). Examine tongue and frenulum under the tongue, soft and hard palate, uvula, and palatoglossal and palatopharyngeal arches in the oral cavity. Photograph with a 35mm camera and colposcopic magnification.

External Genitalia. Explain the procedure to the patient. Position in dorsal lithotomy with legs in padded stirrups. For comfort, obstetric stirrups may be used (Figure 4-13) and the back of the table may be raised (Figure 4-14). Cover the patient's legs and exposed body with warm blankets. Provide rest periods as the patient desires. The advocate may hold her hand if desired and engage the patient in relaxing discussion. Be prepared to collect all specimens before disturbing and manipulating anatomical sites. Video colposcopy, if available, is used for documenting the examination, as well as for teaching and consulting.

Pubic Hair. Place a small paper sheet under the buttocks. Cut matted pubic hair, place in an envelope, and label. Comb the pubic area to collect all possible debris and foreign hairs. Place comb, retrieved hair, and collected debris on the paper sheet. Bindle, package, label, and document. Cut or pull 20 pubic hairs as required by the crime laboratory for the pubic hair standard. The hairs are taken close to the skin and from various places in the pubic area. Bindle, package, label, and document.

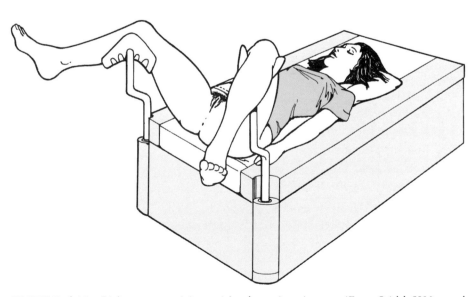

FIGURE 4-13 Lithotomy position with obstetric stirrups. (*From Seidel HM et al:* Mosby's guide to physical examination, *ed 3, St Louis, 1995, Mosby.*)

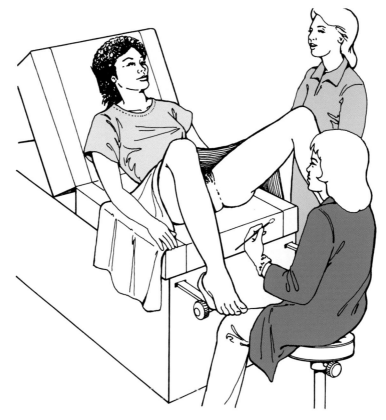

FIGURE 4-14 Lithotomy position with the back elevated. (*From Seidel HM et al:* Mosby's guide to physical examination, *ed 3, St Louis, 1995, Mosby.*)

Examination and Specimen Collection. Inform the patient that you will be touching her genitalia and to let you know about areas that are tender. Lightly palpate the mons veneris and the labia majora, noting areas of tenderness or pain. Use the separation technique of lateral pressure on the labia majora (Figure 4-15). Inspect the sites on the external genitalia (see Figure 1-1) and thighs for foreign material (Figures 4-16 and 4-17) and for injury. Injury may be classified into TEARS (see p. 95).

Follow the standard technique: begin from 12 o'clock and proceed from top to bottom, outside to inside. Use the face of a clock to identify the sites of injury. Injury is most common from 3 o'clock to 9 o'clock when the victim is supine since this is the area where the penis first and most consistently contacts the genitalia. Injury seen without magnification should be recorded as evident by gross visualization. Each injury must be carefully documented with the size, shape, color, location, lesions, secretions, associated pain, and bleeding. Any source of bleeding must be identified. Menstrual bleeding does not exclude secondary source of bleeding that must be identified. A large cotton-tipped applicator may be positioned vaginally to absorb the menstrual bleeding

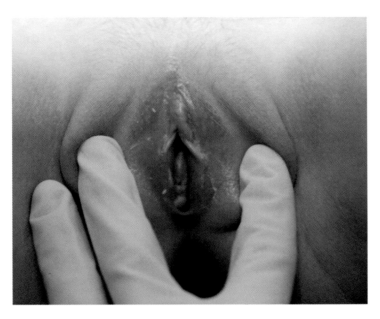

FIGURE 4-15   Separation technique. Examination is 3 hours postassault (35mm). Patient is a white 14 year old, Tanner Stage 2.

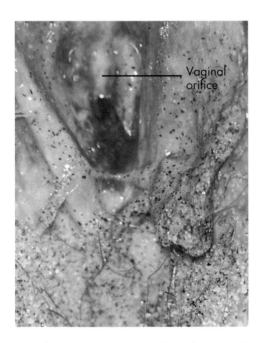

FIGURE 4-16   Foreign material on the genitalia and perineum (sand from an assault that occurred on a beach) (×15).

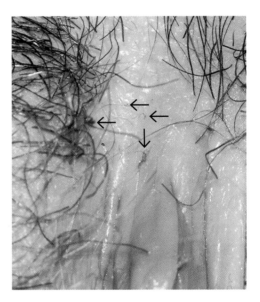

FIGURE 4-17   Foreign material (navy blue fibers on the prepuce of the clitoris) (×15). The blanket on top of which the assault occurred was navy blue.

while examining for injury related sources of bleeding. Culture lesions such as herpes according to local protocol.

Take 35mm photographs, proceeding from wide-to-narrow focus and decreasing-to-increasing magnification (see Photodocumentation, pp. 119-120). Follow with colposcopic magnification to systematically inspect and photograph the external genitalia while maneuvering the anatomical structures to enhance visualization of TEARS.

Toluidine Blue dye 1% is used to highlight lacerations that need to be more clearly visualized (Lauber, Souma, 1982; McCauley and others, 1986). (see Toluidine Blue Dye, pp. 120-121). Photographs at 35mm and with colposcopic magnification should be taken of lacerations seen by gross visualization before both the Toluidine application/decolorization and the digital and speculum examination to substantiate that injury is not caused by this digital and speculum examination. Paint Toluidine Blue dye onto the fossa navicularis and posterior fourchette and extending from 4 o'clock to 8 o'clock (Figure 4-18), where the laceration is present. Decolorize with 10% acetic acid solution or lubricating jelly. Gently blot any excess solution or lubricant.

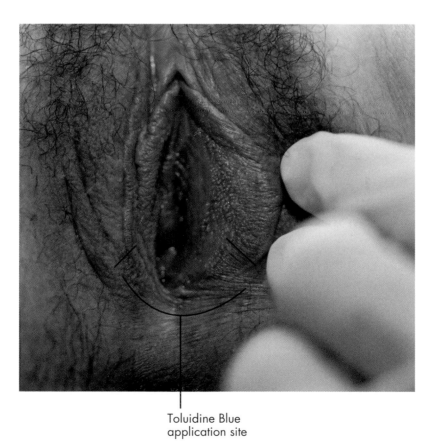

Toluidine Blue
application site

FIGURE 4-18   Toluidine Blue dye application site (×15).

Figures 4-19 to 4-23 are the highlights of an external examination.

Vagina and Cervix. Show the patient the speculum (Figure 4-24), and inform them that first, two fingers will be inserted into the vagina and gently pressed downward, before inserting the speculum. This facilitates speculum insertion and allows for assessment for tenderness and selecting an appropriate speculum size. Figure 4-25 shows the insertion of a vaginal speculum. Lubricate speculum with warm water and not a lubricant. Wait until you feel muscle relaxation. With fingers still in place, insert the closed speculum obliquely and at a 45-degree angle

downward as patient is taking slow deep breaths to facilitate relaxation. Remove fingers and rotate the blades into a horizontal position, maintaining the pressure posteriorly. Open the blades after full insertion and gently maneuver the speculum so the cervix is visualized. On a retroverted uterus, the cervix may be visualized more anteriorly (Seidel and others, 1995). Inspect the vaginal walls and cervix for TEARS and foreign materials.

A pediatric speculum is useful on the sexually inactive adolescent without a menstrual period as well as on some elderly. STDs in adolescents are evaluated from cervical swabs and not vagi-

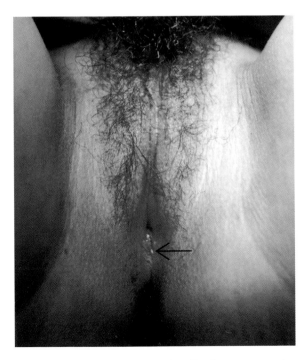

FIGURE 4-19 Gross visualization: posterior fourchette laceration, visible without magnification (35mm). Figures 4-19 through 4-23 are of the same patient.

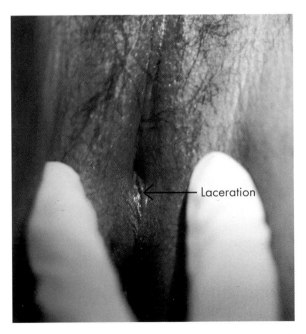

FIGURE 4-20 Posterior fourchette laceration with separation (35mm).

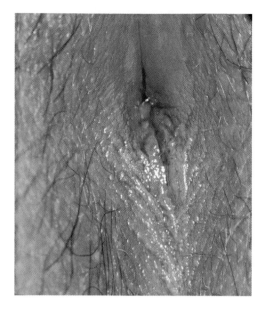

FIGURE 4-21 Posterior fourchette tear (×15).

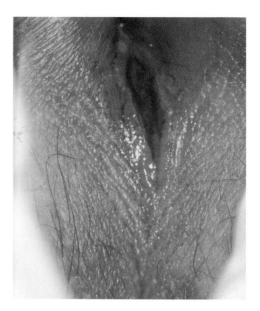

FIGURE 4-22 Posterior fourchette tear using separation technique (×15). Tear is oozing serous fluid.

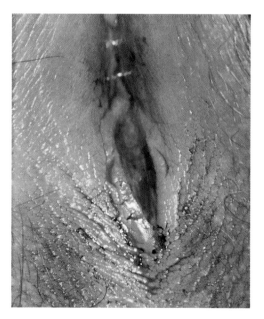

FIGURE 4-23 Posterior fourchette tear after Toluidine Blue dye application/decolorization (×15). Poor dye uptake of an obvious laceration occurred as a result of oozing.

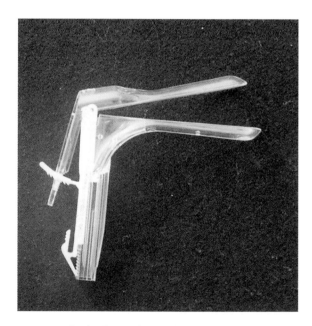

FIGURE 4-24 Vaginal speculum (35mm).

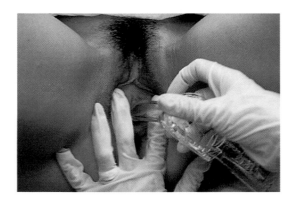
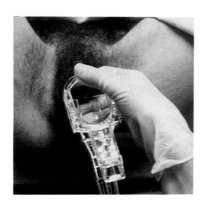
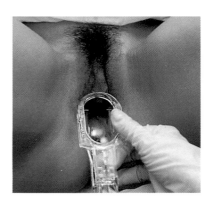
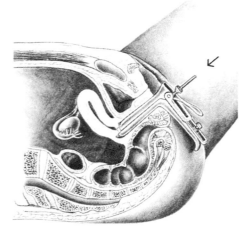
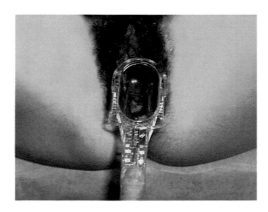
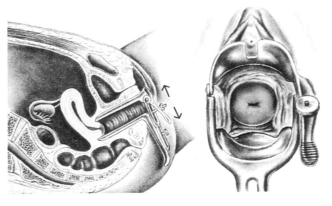

FIGURE 4-25 Insertion of a vaginal speculum (35mm). (*From Seidel HM et al:* Mosby's guide to physical examination, *ed 3, St Louis, 1995, Mosby.*)

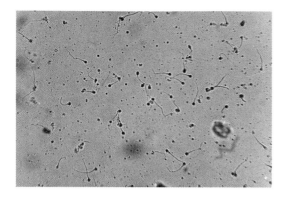

FIGURE 4-26   Microscopic view of spermatozoa (×74).

nal swabs. Referral is necessary for excessive vaginal bleeding or when the source of bleeding cannot be identified.

Collect the following four swabs from the vaginal pool (two deep, two shallow):

Swab 1: Swab the vaginal canal, avoiding the cervix. Prepare a slide using the vaginal swab to make a smear. Moisten the smear with one drop of sterile water (wet-mount). Within 10 minutes of collecting the specimen, check it with a light staining microscope for the presence and motility of spermatozoa (Figure 4-26). Dry, label, and document.

Both the presence and the motility of spermatozoa help corroborate approximately when intercourse occurred. However, there are widely varying rates for clearing of semen from the vagina.

The absence of spermatozoa after vaginal penile intercourse may result from the lack of ejaculation, a vasectomy, or loss of semen before evidence collection. Motile spermatozoa were evident in wet mounts of vaginal smears up to 24 hours after the assault in women up to 49 years of age ($n=29$) but only within 6

hours in postmenopausal women ($n=129$) (Ramin and others, 1992). Sperm retain their motility longer in the cervix, so the source of the specimen must be identified. Nonmotile sperm were detected from vaginal smears in 46% to 71% of women within 72 hours of penile vaginal assault (Dahlke, Cooke, Cunnane, 1977; Jenny and others 1990; Short and others, 1978) and within a considerably longer period in cervical specimens (Soules and others, 1978).

The probability of conception from a single, random, unprotected intercourse is estimated to be between 2% and 4%. When the exposure was midcycle (day 11 to day 18 of a 28-day cycle), the probability of conception is at least 10%, and as high as 30% if exposure was on the day of ovulation (Office of Criminal Justice Planning, 1990). The Committee of the Judiciary of the U.S. Senate (1991) identifies the probability of pregnancy with midcycle exposure as 17%.

The crime laboratory analyzes these swabs for semen markers. High levels of prostatic acid phosphatase, p30 protein, or MHS-5 antigen are conclusive evidence that ejaculation occurred (Herr, Woodward, 1987). Extremely high levels of acid phosphatase are unlikely to be found more than 10 to 12 hours post intercourse (Smally, 1982). Specimens with cells may be processed for DNA typing, which may specifically identify or exclude a potential offender (Thompson, Ford, 1989). DNA fingerprinting of blood, semen, skin, and hair are becoming more widespread, and their results are admissible as evidence in many jurisdictions (Chakraborty, Kidd, 1991).

Swab 2: Collect a second swab from the vaginal wall. Prepare two dry-mount slides. Mark slides with identifying data. Dry swabs and slides. From vaginal swabs or trace evidence, it is possible to identify insoluble lubricant traces such as cornstarch from latex condoms. This identification technique will be increasingly valuable as more perpetrators wear condoms than the 25% that currently do (Blackledge, Vincenti, 1994).

Swab 3 and 4: Collect two swabs from deep in the vagina. Dry, label, and document.

Additional swabs: Collect endocervical swabs and other STD tests as required by the local protocol. Because there is little forensic value in the STD test results in the sexually active population, many agencies treat for potential STDs without culturing. Positive cultures within 72 hours of the assault probably indicate infection that antedated the assault (CDC, 1993) (see Chapter 3). An endocervical swab may also be obtained to examine for spermatozoa, if the assault occurred more than 24 hours before the examination and no possibility exists of a contaminating specimen from a subsequent coitus. Nonmotile spermatozoa may persist in the cervical mucus for up to 17 days (Graves, Sensabaugh, Blake, 1985).

Washings may be collected for the presence of spermatozoa according to the protocol. Following the collection of the swabs, instill 1 to 2 ml of sterile water and catch the secretions in a gauze pad when removing the speculum. This will be examined for the presence of spermatozoa. Dry, label, and document.

If menstrual blood is obscuring inspection of vagina and cervix, use a large swab and position it in the bottom of the vagina. It acts as a tampon to absorb blood. Dry, label, document, then photograph.

Perianal Area. The anus may be examined in the dorsal lithotomy, prone, knee-chest, or lateral decubitus position. Even if the patient denies anal penetration, careful inspection of the area is important.

Examine perineum, anal folds and anus by gently spreading the tissue and observing for TEARS, secretions and foreign material. Gently palpate the anal folds to reveal swelling and tenderness. Photograph with 35mm and colposcopic magnification. Photographs before the anoscopic examination substantiate that the significant findings antedated the anoscope insertion. Collect all debris and dried secretions.

If indicated by the history or presence of perianal TEARS, prepare to collect anal swabs by first cleaning the perianal area to prevent contamination from vaginal secretions. Dilate anus using anal speculum. Then, sequentially collect two anal swabs, just inside the anus and prepare two dry mount slides. If indicated and within 6 hours postassault, prepare a wet-mount of smear for the microscopic detection of spermatozoa. Collect swabs for STD testing, as required by the local protocol. Dry, label, and document. There is rapid deterioration of sexual products in the anus and rectum as a result of the bacterial concentration, so specimens should be obtained in a timely fashion.

Toluidine Blue dye may be used to highlight lacerations, after specimens have been obtained and before the anoscopic examination. When 35 mm and colposcopic photographs clearly identify the injury, Toluidine Blue dye may not be necessary. When used, Toluidine Blue dye is swabbed onto the perianal area. Then the dye is decolorized with a 10% acetic acid or lubricating jelly. Blot the excess. Photograph and document.

Anoscopic Examination. Perform the anoscopic examination if the history indicates that anal contact or penetration has occurred or if there are perianal findings. Some patients may be too embarrassed to affirm anal contact or penetration, or they are unable to recall the details of the incident, which may result in a negative history with positive findings. Conversely, there may be a history positive for anal penetration with no physical findings, since 50% of the patients with anal penetration have no findings (Greene, 1996).

The clear lubricated anoscope (Figure 4-27) is gently inserted to the flange as the patient continues breathing slowly. Remove the obturator, hold the anoscope securely and begin inspecting for TEARS. Inspect and take colposcopic photographs at three levels: (1) with anoscope inserted completely (Figure 4-28), (2) halfway out (Figure 4-29), and (3) just before removing the anoscope (Figure 4-30). Remove the anoscope.

If perianal area is too tender for anoscopic examination, try the knee-chest position to help relax the sensitive sphincter. If still unable to proceed, and specimens have been obtained, topical lidocaine (Xylocaine) may be used. Least preferred is for the patient to return the next day for the examination. Remind the patient

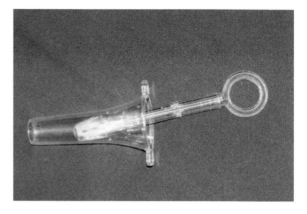

FIGURE 4-27   Anoscope (35mm).

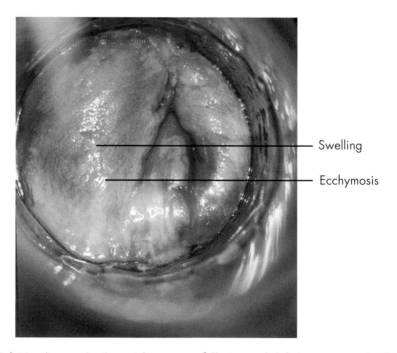

FIGURE 4-28   Anoscopic view with anoscope fully inserted; lubricant was used (×15). There is swelling and bruising. Figures 4-28 to 4-30 are of the same patient, a 28-year-old male who was abducted and sodomized in the backseat of a car.

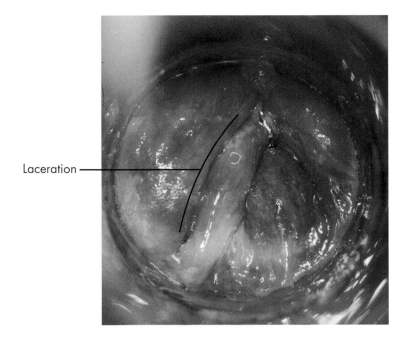

Laceration ——

FIGURE 4-29 Anoscope halfway out (×15). A laceration at 7 o'clock extending to 1 o'clock.

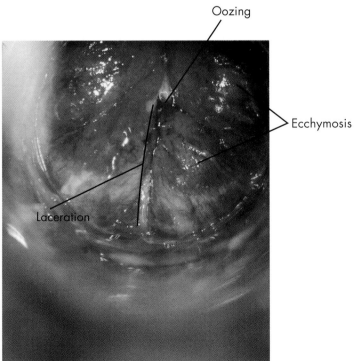

Oozing

Ecchymosis

Laceration

FIGURE 4-30 Anoscope just beyond the anal orifice (×15). There is a laceration from 6 o'clock, extending centrally. The central end of the laceration is oozing blood. There is ecchymosis at 2 o'clock and 4 o'clock.

how vital it is to identify, document, and photograph the findings.

Techniques for the Examination of Adolescent and Elderly Females

Understanding the developmental characteristics of adolescent and elderly patients may help the examiner modify techniques for the history and physical examination, specifically to those patient groups.

The adolescent

Adolescent physical development may range from Stages 1 to 5 on Tanner's Scale (1962) (Table 4-2). Typically, adolescents 13 to 18 years old are Tanner Stage 3, 4, or 5. However, in the adolescent that is Stage 1 or 2, recall that the unestrogenized hymen is sensitive and a speculum examination may be painful. The adolescent may be either sexually naïve or sexually experienced. Adolescence is a time form asserting independence, separating from authority figures, emancipating from parents, attaching to peers, preparing for careers, and taking risks (Gilchrist, 1991). Understanding these developmental characteristics helps the examiner anticipate the needs of the adolescent patient during the examination.

Beginning the history with an open-ended question such as, "Tell me what happened," may be helpful in determining the experience, values, and language that the adolescent uses. If the perpetrator is a family member of the adolescent, child abuse reporting laws must be considered before agreeing to maintain confidentiality. Examination techniques for adolescents are listed in left and middle columns of the box on pp. 114-115.

The elderly

The elderly may be hesitant to give a sexual history, refer to sexual body parts, describe the sexual contact, and quote terms the perpetrator used in describing the assault. Their perceptions about sexual intimacy were formed in more traditional times, as a victim of sexual assault, they may experience overwhelming shame and guilt. They may be more modest and stoic than the younger patient.

The history for the elderly must include a sexual history. The examiner should ask about the year of their last period, any estrogen therapy, frequency of sexual intercourse and/or manual genital stimulation, and pain or bleeding with sexual intercourse. Medical conditions such as previous multiparity, diabetes mellitus, genital trauma, surgery, or unattended births must be documented if they may affect the examination and the findings. Many elderly females have physical problems that may interfere with their sexual activity. A patient who experiences painful joints, dyspnea, or fear of causing illness or injury is less likely to engage in consensual sexual intercourse. This information may be useful to clarify whether the reported act was likely to be consensual. Additional examination techniques for the elderly are listed in the middle and right columns of Box 4-2, pp. 114-115.

Techniques for the Examination of Male Patients

The most common forms of sexual assault in males is receptive anal and oral intercourse, as well as genital manipulation of the patient (Hillman, 1992). Therefore the anus, mouth, and genitalia are the focus of the physical examination of the male patient.

The male patient may feel guilty about having been assaulted because males are supposed to be able to protect themselves. The examiner may inform them that many patients are immobilized by the incident and are unable to re-

Table 4-2	*Sexual Development in the Female*	
STAGE	PUBIC HAIR	BREASTS
1	Preadolescent; only fine vellus hair similar to that on the abdomen	Preadolescent; elevation of nipple only
2	Sparse growth of long, slightly pigmented downy hair—straight or slightly curled—along the labia	Breast bud stage Elevation of breast and nipple as a small mound; enlargement of areolar diameter

Continued.

Table 4-2	*Sexual Development in the Female—cont'd*	
STAGE	PUBIC HAIR	BREASTS
3	Darker, coarser, curlier hair, spreading sparsely over the labia	Further enlargement and elevation of breast and areola No separation of their contours
	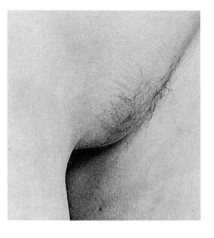	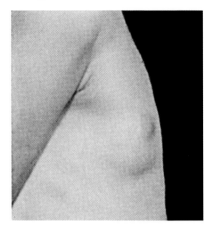
4	Coarse and curly as in adults Area covered is greater than Stage 3, and not yet adult in extent	Projection of areola and nipple to form a secondary mound above the level of the breast
	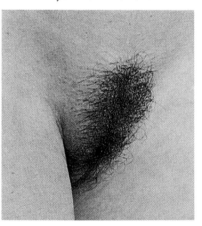	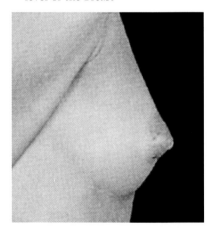

Table 4-2	*Sexual Development in the Female—cont'd*	
STAGE	PUBIC HAIR	BREASTS
5	Quality and quantity of hair is adult pattern Spread on medial surface of thighs	Mature stage Areola recedes to same contour as breast and is strongly pigmented; some still have secondary mound

Adapted from Seidel HM and others: *Mosby's guide to physical examination*, ed 3, St Louis, 1995, Mosby; Tanner JM: Growth at adolescence, ed 2, Oxford, 1962, Blackwell Scientific. Illustrations from Van Wieringen JC: *Growth diagrams, 1965 Netherlands Second national survey on 0-24-year-olds*, Groningen, Netherlands, 1971, Wolters-Noordhoff; reprinted with permission from Kluwer Academic Publishers.

sist. Encourage them to verbalize their reactions and fears. Explain that it is a common misunderstanding that sexually assaulted men become homosexual from the assault. The patient is in the acute phase of rape trauma syndrome (see p. 84) and may respond in an expressed or controlled style. Typically, male victims are more controlled, sullen, and withdrawn. Adolescent males who are asserting their independence, being influenced by peers, taking risks, and defending those risks expect no one to understand their situation and may have difficulty reaching out and accepting support.

In preparation for the history and examination, ask them about themselves, not just about the assault. Explain what is done during the examination and why it is done using their terms and at their developmental level. Offer possible choices, abiding by the choice made. This helps to return some control to the patient. Offer a male or female advocate. Ledray (1992) found that males prefer female care providers because male providers symbolize the perpetrator. Give examples of other adolescents to whom this has happened. Help him envision positive possibilities for coping with the assault and facilitate his decision making. Let him know that the advocate is available for him, even in court.

History and Physical Examination of the Adult and Adolescent Male

Avoid leaving blanks on the examination form by marking "not applicable" (n/a) on the sections of the form that refer to female anatomy, and feminine hygiene products. The examiner may need to begin the interview by saying, "Many rapists do all kinds of things to

Box 4-2	*Examination Techniques for Adolescent and Elderly Females*	
ADOLESCENT	**ADOLESCENT AND ELDERLY**	**ELDERLY**

ADOLESCENT

- Face the adolescent
- Be aware that parents may feel suspect
- Do not talk down to the patient
- Reporting is required by law for child abuse cases
- Ask what the adolescent prefers to keep confidential from parent
- Allow adolescent to decide if parent should be present during the history
- Adolescent can consent to testing and prescription for STD without parent consent or knowledge (CDC, 1993)
- Excuse parent before the speculum examination; this increases cooperation (Carson, 1992)
- Most prefer no chaperone during *routine* pelvic examination (Carson, 1992)
- Determine Tanner stage (see Table 4-2)
- Provide accurate information about body parts
- Reassure that examination will not tear her hymen
- Encourage her to help with her examination by holding her legs, positioning the scale or pressing the shutter for photos
- Alternate positioning supine holding her knees, with lithotomy position
- Perform labial traction on the unestrogenized adolescent to examine the vaginal walls; speculum examination in an unestrogenized hymen is painful

ADOLESCENT AND ELDERLY

- Ask about sexual history
- Use age appropriate terms
- May need to wait for an answer to examiner questions
- Ask if needs more time or more explanation. Avoid saying "do you understand?"
- Use speculum of appropriate size based on visualization of introitus
- Use eye contact
- Direct her to void before the pelvic examination
- Begin to examine nongenital areas before genital areas
- Show her the speculum and/or let her manipulate it
- Ask what her experience has been with previous speculum examinations
- Explain what you will do before each step
- Gently insert two fingers vaginally, look to evaluate tolerance for speculum
- Use models and diagrams to explain
- Reassure her that the perpetrator was wrong, not her
- Explain that her foggy memory is normal
- Avoid saying the following:
  "This won't hurt."
  "It could have been worse."
  "What did you expect?"
  "Were you a virgin before?"
  "Why didn't you fight?"
  "Don't you feel some pain here?"
  . . . and other leading questions
- Avoid showing surprise or disgust

ELDERLY

- Anticipate more hesitancy in giving a sexual history, referring to body parts and using terms the perpetrator may have used
- Ask about hip and leg pain, which may occur during lithotomy positioning, as well as discomforts during last pap smear
- List medications used
- Ask specifically about abstinence and if it results from shortness of breath, pain, and others
- Ask about gynecological surgeries and her use of the estrogen that may be prescribed
- Elevate head slightly
- Try supporting calves on padded stirrups or using obstetric stirrups (see Figure 4-13)
- Offer repositioning every 30 minutes while in lithotomy position
- Offer warm blanket even during the history. Offer socks and warm blankets during examination
- Drape for modesty
- Anticipate that the Introitus may be small or gape open
- Consider pediatric specula
- Inquire about vaginal wall tenderness, especially if bleeding or pain
- Be prepared for the potential for vaginal or cervical bleeding resulting from friable tissue
- Differentiate vaginal atrophy from atrophic or senile vaginitis
- Wet swab with sterile water when taking vaginal swabs, if vagina is dry

Box 4-2	*Examination Techniques for Adolescent and Elderly Females—cont'd*	
ADOLESCENT	**ADOLESCENT AND ELDERLY**	**ELDERLY**
• Perform a speculum examination on estrogenized adolescent with reported vaginal penetration (Heger, Emans, 1992). • Use the smallest speculum, Huffman (1/2″ x 4 1/4″) for the sexually inactive adolescent; use a Pederson (7/8″ x 4 1/2″) for the sexually active adolescent (Heger, Emans, 1992) • Be prepared to observe normal cervical ectropian in one third of pubertal girls (Rimsza, 1989), redundant hymen, and vestibular papillations • Teach about contraception and STDs		• Swab from the vaginal pool if no cervix

their victims. What was your experience?" Avoid questions suggesting specific facts that may have occurred.

The principles of control, dry, package, label, and document apply to evidence collected from the male examination. Explain the equipment and what will be done, and give him the opportunity to assist with the examination, such as with positioning, holding the scale, retracting for photographs, and pressing the shutter release button to take the photos. Injuries should be diagramed and photographed with 35mm and colposcopic magnification. Teach as you move through the examination, especially describing the sensations that might be felt (i.e., "This dye might feel cool."). Start with the Wood's lamp or alternative light source to examine his clothes. Document the location on the clothing that fluoresces. Package, label, and document.

The male genitalia are examined with the patient in a supine, sitting, or standing position (Figure 4-31). The Tanner Stages of Sexual Development of the Male are identified (Table 4-3). Examine the thighs, penis, scrotum, and perineum for TEARS, bite marks, secretions, and discharge. Have the patient retract his foreskin. Use a Wood's lamp or alternative light source on his body, genitalia, and perianal area. Swab the secretions, fluorescing body sites, bite marks, and where it is reported that the perpetrator had oral contact. Dry, label, and document, including the location of specimen. Obtain a control; dry and label.

Wet two swabs with sterile water and swab the urethral orifice for chlamydia and gonorrhea, according to protocol for culturing for STDs. With the second swab, swab the glans penis and shaft. Obtain a dry-mount culture for herpetic lesions per protocol.

For the perianal examination, position the male patient supine holding his knees on his chest, laterally or standing, while bent over the examination table. Insure that the colposcope reaches. Either the patient or examiner can spread the buttocks. The perianal and anoscopic examination is conducted in the male patient as is described in the female examination (see pp. 107-110).

Special Techniques

Anterior labial traction

This is a technique to improve visualization of the hymen and vaginal mucosa. This technique is useful for examining the vaginal walls in the nonestrogenized female when the speculum examination is painful and unnecessary in most cases of sexual assault (Heger, Emans, 1992). Most foreign bodies are visible with this method, and deep vaginal swabs are more easily obtained when speculum examination is not used. To perform the examination, firmly grasp both labia majora (not the minora) with the thumb and index finger of each hand, then gently but firmly pull the labia forward and slightly to the side.

Balloon-covered swab

A blue or green balloon on the end of a swab is inserted vaginally just beyond the hymen (Figure 4-32). The swab is used to flatten out the hymenal folds. The color contrast helps evaluate the continuity of the edges of the hymen.

Castings of bite marks

The American Society of Forensic Odontology recommends the protocol for taking the

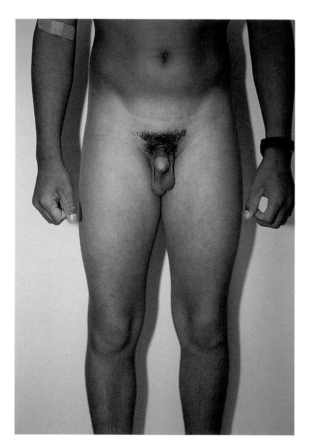

FIGURE 4-31 Male examination performed with patient standing (35mm). Patient is a Hispanic 14 year old, Tanner Stage 4, assaulted rectally and orally.

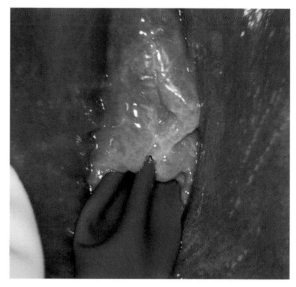

FIGURE 4-32 Balloon-covered swab technique (×15). Notches are at 12 o'clock and 2 o'clock, which in the child, may be congenital remnants or may result from healed lacerations. (*From Heger A, Emans SJ, editors:* Evaluation of the sexually abused child, *New York, 1992, Oxford University Press*).

Table 4-3 *Sexual Development in the Male*		
STAGE	PUBIC HAIR	PENIS, TESTES AND SCROTUM
1	Preadolescent; only fine vellus hair like that on the abdomen	Preadolsecent; same proportions as in childhood
2	Sparse growth of long, slightly pigmented, downy hair, straight or slightly curled, mostly at the base of the penis	Slight or no enlargement of penis; testes and scrotum larger; scrotum reddened
3	Darker, coarser, curlier hair spreading sparsely over the symphysis	Further enlargement of testes and penis in length; descent of scrotum.

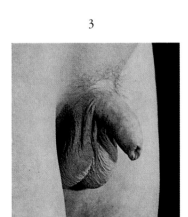

Continued.

Table 4-3	*Sexual Development in the Male—cont'd*		
STAGE	PUBIC HAIR		PENIS, TESTES AND SCROTUM
4	Pigmented, coarse, and curly hair, as in the adult; area covered is greater than in Stage 3 but not extending to the adult pattern		Further enlarged; scrotal skin darkened
5	Adult size and shape; spreading to medial thighs.		Adult size and shape; scrotum ample; penis reaches almost to the bottom of the scrotum

Adapted from Seidel HM and others: *Mosby's guide to physical examination,* ed. 3, St Louis, 1995, Mosby; Tanner JM: *Growth at adolescence,* ed 2, Oxford, 1962, Blackwell Scientific. Illustrations from Van Wieringen JC: *Growth diagrams, 1965 Netherlands Second national survey on 0-24-year-olds,* Groningen, Netherlands, 1971, Wolters-Noordhoff; reprinted with permission from Kluwer Academic Publishers.

casting of bite marks that have left an indentation. (Bowers, Bell, 1995) If the marks are flush with the skin surface, castings are not indicated.

Load a delivery syringe such as polysulfide rubber base syringe or static mixing syringe with polyvinyl siloxane or polyether impression material. Inject it over the bitemark keeping the material "gap-free" to minimize air trapping. Place orthopedic (e.g., Hexcelite) tape onto the setting material and then spread more material on top of the tape, thus creating a "sandwich" of impression material with the tape in the middle. You can reinforce this later with quick-set plaster. The Hexcelite can mold to curved surfaces when placed in hot water.

Colposcopy

Colposcopy provides binocular vision, with magnification from 5 to 30 times, and the ability to take photographs (Figure 4-33). Magnification of 15 times is commonly used. Video camera recording may also be a feature.

In a study by Slaughter and Brown (1992) the identification of injury was 87% with colposcopic magnification, compared with 10% to 30% without colposcopy. The improved identification of injury with magnification was also found in a study of injury in consensual intercourse (Norvell, Benrubi, and Thompson, 1984). Hand-held magnifiers do not have the photographic capability of colposcopy, but are a useful aid to examine for injury.

Foley catheter

Figure 4-34 shows a Foley with a 5 ml balloon inserted to just beyond the hymen. The Foley is inflated with 40 to 50 ml of air and gently pulled downward. It improves the examination of the hymen (Ferrell, 1995).

Photodocumentation

Photographs (35mm and colposcopic magnification), taken systematically, of each of the injuries support the physical examination findings for the record, and are useful for teaching, consultation, and legal proceedings. Not photographing injuries, wounds, trauma, and abuse may open the examiner to liability and negligence for failure to adequately document (Pasqualone, 1996). See Colposcopy, above, for a description of magnification.

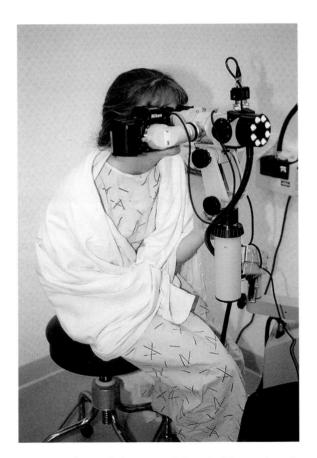

FIGURE 4-33 Colposcope (35mm). The patient is looking through the opticals of the colposcope after her examination. A camera is mounted on the right side of the colposcope.

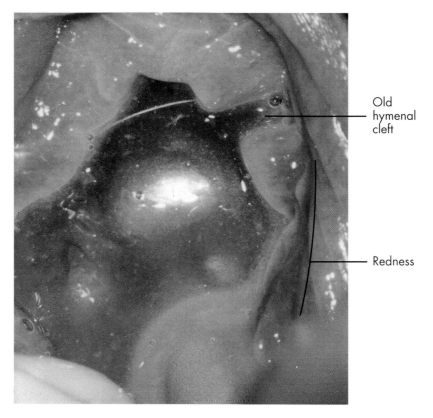

Old hymenal cleft

Redness

FIGURE 4-34   Foley balloon technique shows an old hymenal cleft at 2 o'clock. Hymen is red from 3 o'clock to 5 o'clock on this white, sexually active 15 year old (×15).

For the best photographs, use a 35mm camera and macro lens, 60mm to 105mm with 1:1 ratio continuous focusing. The macro lens allows for close-up photographs. An instant photograph does not give the quality of emulsion needed. A tripod with a bayonet arm allows for photos 90 degrees from the injury, which helps eliminate distortion. Take a photograph of the same site without the photomacrographic scale to document the area obscured by the scale. Photos on blue backdrop give better skin color. Use a databack to get the date, time, and case number on the frame (Golden, 1996). If there is no databack, include the patient's record number, date, and time on a self-sticking note attached to the photomacrographic scale used in the photograph. Less desirable is to label with the date, time, and case number immediately after development.

Take photos from top to bottom and outside to inside with a wide-to-narrow focus and decreasing-to-increasing magnification. Take two photos of each finding. Use a photographic review sheet to record each photo. Review and make your own notes concerning the photos promptly after their development.

Toluidine Blue dye

One percent aqueous solution dyes nucleate squamous cells in the deeper layers of the epi-

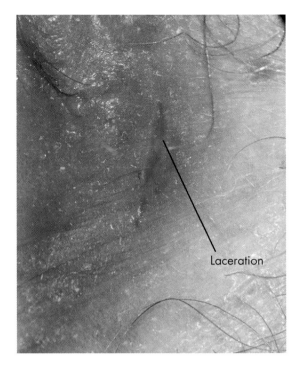

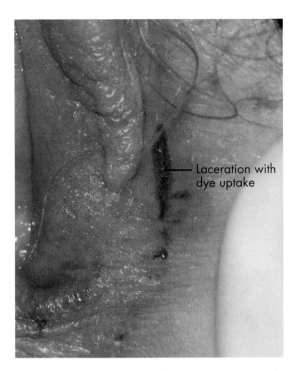

FIGURE 4-35   Laceration before Toluidine Blue dye (×15). Figures 4-35 and 4-36 are the same patient. The laceration is on the left labium major, clearly visible. This is a white 16 year old who was penetrated vaginally twice with the penis and six times digitally while she was bent over a cabinet.

FIGURE 4-36   Laceration after Toluidine Blue dye. There is distinct dye uptake (×15). Redness is generalized.

dermis exposed by lacerations. Toluidine Blue dye should be used to highlight lacerations that are seen by colposcopy and should not be used as a screening method (Slaughter, Brown, 1992). Deep blue uptake is interpreted as positive for laceration injury. Figures 4-35 and 4-36 show a laceration before and after Toluidine Blue dye application. No uptake or diffuse uptake (Figure 4-37) is negative for laceration. Diffuse uptake may occur in inflammation such as vulvitis (Lauber, Souma, 1982). The dye is not to be used on mucous membranes because the uptake will be diffuse and nonspecific for laceration.

Toluidine Blue dye does not discolor intact keratinized skin. Toluidine and destaining

reagents do not affect DNA profiles from vaginal swabs (Hochmeister and others, 1996). Toluidine Blue dye is spermicidal in vitro but has not been shown to affect acid phosphatase levels (Lauber, Souma, 1982). Toluidine Blue does not highlight old episiotomy scars. It has improved the detection of injury in adolescents and children and dark-skinned patients (McCauley and others, 1986).

In a group of 24 assaulted females, posterior fourchette lacerations were identified by gross visualization in 4% of the females. When Toluidine dye was applied, lacerations were evident in 54% of those same females (McCauley and others, 1986). Superficial lacerations may otherwise be difficult to demonstrate because of the rugations in the posterior fourchette.

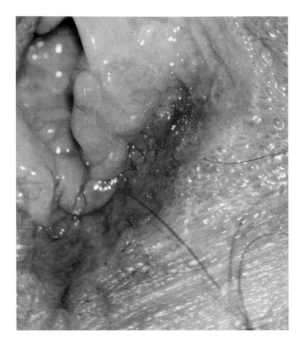

FIGURE 4-37 Diffuse Toluidine Blue dye: negative for laceration (×15).

Wood's lamp and alternative light source

The ultraviolet light (see Figure 4-7) of the Wood's lamp is capable of fluorescing semen stains, as well as substances like detergents and certain clothing fibers (Secofsky, 1996). It is best used in a darkened room. Inform them that you will darken the room, then shine the lamp on a nondigital watch or other fluorescing substance to show what you are trying to find.

The alternative light source is a 450 nm visible blue light. As it illuminates the skin, augmentation may appear as patterned injuries such as bruises and bite marks when viewed through color-blocking filters. The light is absorbed by hematological components in the injury, and the surrounding dermal tissue fluoresces, augmenting the appearance of marks (Golden, 1994). Saliva, semen, vaginal fluid, and blood may also be detected (Golden, 1996).

CONCLUDE

Concluding the Initial Examination

In concluding the initial examination, the examiner teaches, treats, connects, and checks. Written instructions are necessary since patients' recall may be reduced from the stress of the incident (Kramer and others, 1991).

Teach

Provide a concise and readable handout of important points (see Appendix C). Patient objectives are to do the following:

1. Understand examination findings, follow-up care, and the necessity for the follow-up examination. Make an appointment for a follow-up examination with the forensic examiner.

2. Make another appointment with a routine health care provider for hepatitis B immune globulin (HBIG) within 14 days of exposure to HBV through sexual contact with a person who has acute or chronic HBV infection. Also begin the HBV vaccination series at time of examination, 1, and 6 months (CDC, 1993). Plan for HIV testing at 3 and 6 months.

3. Take medications until completed and monitor for side effects such as nausea following norgestrel (Ovral). Understand the use of a condom for intercourse until medications are completed. If single-dose antibiotics were given, condoms should still be used for at least 7 days (CDC, 1996). Provide a handout for the correct use of a condom (CDC, 1993).

4. Avoid sexual intercourse with partners infected with STDs.

5. Soak perineum in warm water twice daily for comfort and to facilitate healing. Assume hygienic care.

6. Eat yogurt with active cultures to help avoid

antibiotic-induced diarrhea and drink cranberry juice to help avoid urinary tract infection (UTI).

7. Anticipate feelings that may occur following sexual assault, such as rape trauma syndrome (Burgess, Hartman, 1995). The examiner should discuss these feelings briefly as well as relevant myths of sexual assault (see Appendix A) as the handout is reviewed.

8. Know relaxation techniques and use visual imagery. Identify a support person in whom to confide. Refer to counseling (see Connect, below, right).

9. Understand that reporting the incident is different than prosecuting the perpetrator. Victim services can answer questions about legal, judicial, medical, and financial supports.

Treat

For sexually transmitted diseases, prophylactic drug treatment may be offered at the time of the examination rather than waiting for test results. Prophylactic drug treatment is indicated because (1) initial cultures may be negative, but the patient may have been exposed to infection; (2) nearly 50% fail to return for follow-up care (Jenny and others, 1990), so disease control is enhanced by prophylactic treatment; and (3) many patients are reassured to have preventive treatment.

Follow current CDC guidelines for STDs and sexual assault. See Chapter 3 for further explanation of infection associated with sexual assault. CDC (1993) recommends treatment for the following potential STDs and pregnancy:

- *Gonorrhea:* Ceftriaxone (Rocephin) 125 mg or 250 mg intramuscularly, in a single dose
- *Chlamydia:* Doxycycline (Doxy 100) 100 mg orally, twice daily for 7 days, or azithromycin (Zithromax) 1 gm by mouth in a single dose. If less than 15 years old, doxycycline is acceptable, but the safety in using azithromycin for that age group has not yet been established. In pregnancy, use erythromycin base (E-base) 500 mg by mouth, four times daily for 7 days
- *Trichomoniasis and bacterial vaginosis:* Metronidazole (Flagyl) 500 mg twice daily for 7 days or 2 gm by mouth, in a single dose.
- *Hepatitis B vaccine:* Three doses: at time of examination, 1 month, and 6 months. The use of HBIG, combined with vaccination, can prevent infection among persons exposed sexually to HBV if administered within 14 days of exposure (CDC, 1993).
- *Pregnancy:* If the pregnancy test is negative and within 3 days of the assault, offer norgestrel (Ovral), two tabs at time of examination and 2 tabs in 12 hours. Take with promethazine (Phenergan) 25 mg by mouth every 4 to 6 hours as needed for nausea.

Connect

Review with victim services before leaving the examination facility (Burgess and others, 1995). The advocate may serve as the liaison to victim services in some centers. Victim services help patients understand and access available financial, legal, medical, social, and counseling support. Appendix C is a model of a patient information form. It includes local rape crisis or rape counseling services, as well as the telephone numbers, hours of availability, and languages spoken. The advocate can help access family members or friends for transportation to a safe location and can provide companionship during the initial hours following the assault.

Emphasize that recovery is best with counseling. Counselors should be chosen for their expe-

Box 4-3 *Evidentiary and Reference Samples*	
EVIDENTIARY ITEMS	REFERENCE SAMPLES
Oral swab (2)	Blood tubes
Oral smear	Saliva for secretor status
Vaginal swabs (4)	Head hairs
Vaginal smears (2)	Pubic hairs
Vaginal washing (optional)	Other body hair (e.g., mustache, beard)
Rectal swabs (2)	Urine for toxicology, pregnancy, *and* spermatozoa
Rectal smear	
Pubic hair combings	
Additional swabs (e.g., semen stains, bite marks)	
Nail scrapings and clippings	
Trace evidence (e.g., hairs, fibers, debris)	
Penile swab	
Meatus swab	

rience and expertise in the care of patients who have been sexually assaulted. Rape crisis centers are resources for finding experienced counselors See Appendix B for additional resources. Connect with law enforcement by ensuring that the patient has the telephone number of the officer or detective on the case.

Check

Package all dried evidence, and complete and check labels. Evidentiary items and reference samples to be checked, labeled, and documented are listed in the box above.

Insert all evidence into the crime laboratory box or large envelope and seal. Seal should include the date, time, and initials of the examiner. Store evidence in a locked refrigerator until law enforcement can deliver it to the crime laboratory. Laboratory specimens for culture and pregnancy determination are processed by a local medical laboratory and are not sent with the evidence to the crime laboratory. Cultures and pregnancy tests are not refrigerated.

Complete the chain of custody form, which should include case number, item number, description, person submitting the evidence, person receiving the evidence and the date the evidence was received (ASTM, 1992).

Document on the examination form. List findings and specimens obtained, then summarize, and sign the examination form. The summary concludes with whether the findings are consistent with the history and timing of the reported incident and whether there was evidence of sexual contact (Hampton, 1995; Slaughter, Brown, 1991).

Prepare film for processing. Care should be taken to ensure that the film is correctly identified with the patient's medical record number. Film should be recorded on the chain of custody form. Film may be developed by an experienced commercial photographic laboratory (OCJP, 1990). The laboratory must understand the forensic and sensitive nature of the photos and agree to provide for the proper handling and security of the photographs. A responsible person should deliver the photographic material. Once developed, the photographs should be evaluated, and findings should be noted on the photographic review sheet and organized with the negatives. Avoid marking on the front or backs of the photographs. Photographs should then be filed in a locked cabinet with the medical record.

CONTINUE

The Follow-Up Examination

The follow-up examination has several purposes—to examine for physical healing, infection control and emotional status, to provide and reinforce teaching, and to refer for further care.

Examine

Findings from the 2-week follow-up examination are an essential part of the care of the patient. Acute injury is differentiated from normal variations or other conditions by comparing the findings and photographs of the two examinations. In 2 weeks, the physical evaluation should reveal healing of both genital and nongenital injury. Before the examination, review photos from the initial examination to ensure that positioning and separation techniques are similar. In this way, initial photos and the photos at 2 weeks can most easily be compared. Photos of healing injuries are taken with 35mm and magnification. Appendix F is an example of a follow-up examination form.

A follow-up at 2 weeks also allows for the completion of the medication for STDs (CDC, 1993). If antibiotics were not provided at the initial examination, then STD cultures are indicated for *N. gonorrhea, C. trachomatis,* and *T. vaginalis,* and blood is drawn for *T. pallidum* (CDC, 1993).

Teach

Patients are reminded to continue their HBV series at 1 and 6 months after their initial vaccinations. This may be obtained by their routine health care providers. HIV testing may also be obtained at 3 and 6 months (CDC, 1993).

Emphasize that it is critical to seek out and/or continue counseling because most of those who have been sexually assaulted have some degree of rape trauma syndrome (Burgess and others, 1995). Counseling may help prevent some of the results of having been sexually assaulted, such as difficulties in intimate relationships, sexual dysfunction, difficulty parenting, and a higher tendency to enter relationships in which they are revictimized (Burgess, Hartman, 1995).

Teaching includes explaining the healing of injuries, reviewing measures to avoid revictimization, answering questions about HIV, HBV, and other STDs, and clarifying relevant myths (see Appendix A). More general health care teaching concerns birth control measures, including proper use of a condom (CDC, 1993), annual Pap smears, and monthly breast self-examination.

Refer

Referrals are made for continued health care as indicated. The 12-week follow-up may be conducted by the routine health care provider because there is typically no forensic evidence sought then. At 12 weeks postassault, the CDC (1993) recommends testing for HIV and syphilis if antibiotics were not taken. The 6 months postassault follow-up will include HIV testing and completion of the HBV vaccination series.

REFERENCES

Adams JA, Knudson S: Genital findings in adolescent girls referred for suspected sexual abuse, *Arch Pediatr Adolesc Med* 150:850, 1996.

American Psychiatric Association: Posttraumatic stress disorder. In *Diagnostic and statistical manual of mental disorders,* ed 4, Washington DC, 1994, the Association.

Association for Standards of Testing Materials (ASTM): Standard practice for receiving, documenting, storing and retrieving evidence in a forensic science laboratory, *Annual book of ASTM standards,* Washington, DC, 1992, the Association.

Blackledge RD, Vincenti M: Identification of polydimethyl-siloxane lubricant traces from latex condoms in cases of sexual assault, *J Forens Sci Society* 34:245, 1994.

Bowers CM, Bell G, editors: *Manual of forensic odontology,* City, ST, 1995, American Society of Forensic Odontology.

Burgess AW and others: Victim care services and the comprehensive sexual assault assessment tool. In Hazelwood RR and Burgess AW, editors: *Practical aspects of rape investigation,* Boca Raton, Fla, 1995, CRC Press.

Burgess AW, Fehder W, Hartman C: Delayed reporting of the rape victim, *J Psychsoc Nur* 33:21, 1995.

Burgess AW, Hartman CR: Rape trauma and post traumatic stress disorder. In McBride A, Austin J, editors: *Psychiatric nursing integrating the behavioral and biological sciences,* Philadelphia, 1995, WB Saunders.

Carson SA: Gynecologic examination of the adolescent. In Carpenter SE, Rock J, editors: *Pediatric and adolescent gynecology,* New York, 1992, Raven.

Centers for Disease Control and Prevention: *Personal communication,* November 1996.

Centers for Disease Control and Prevention: Sexually transmitted diseases-treatment guidelines, *MMWR* 42: Atlanta, 1993, US Department of Health and Human Services.

Committee on the Judiciary, US Senate: *Violence against women: the increase in rape in America 1990,* Washington DC, 1991, Library of Congress.

Chakraborty R, Kidd KK: The utility of DNA typing in forensic work, *Science* 254:1735, 1991.

Dahlke MB, Cooke C, Cunnane M: Identification of semen in 500 patients seen because of rape, *Am J Clin Pathol* 68:740, 1977.

Federal Bureau of Investigation: *Uniform crime reports for the United States,* Washington, DC 1993, US Bureau of Justice.

Ferrell J: Foley catheter balloon technique for visualizing the hymen in female adolescent sexual abuse victim, *J Emerg Nurs* 21:585, 1995.

Gilchrist VJ: Preventive health care for the adolescent, *Am Fam Phys* 43:1, 1991.

Golden GC: *Personal communication,* March 1996.

Golden GS: Use of alternative light source illumination in bite mark photography, *J Foren Sci* 39:815, 1994.

Graves HC, Sensabaugh GF, Blake ET: Postcoital detection of male-specific semen protein: application to the investigation of rape, *N Engl J Med* 312:338, 1985.

Greene J: Genital-anal trauma secondary to sexual assault. Paper presented at Naval Hospital, San Diego, Calif, January 1996.

Hampton HL: Care of the woman who has been raped, *N Engl J Med* 332:234, 1995.

Hartman CR, Burgess AW: Rape trauma and treatment of the victim. In Ochberg FM, editor *Post-traumatic therapy and victims of violence,* New York, 1988, Brunner/Mazel.

Heger A, Emans SJ, editors: *Evaluation of the sexually abused child,* New York, 1992, Oxford University Press.

Herr JC, Woodward MP: An enzyme linked immunosorbent assay (ELISA) for human semen identification based on bi-olinylated monoclonal antibody to a seminal vesicle-specific antigen, *J Forens Sci* 32:346, 1987.

Hillman R: Male victims of sexual assault, *Brit J Gen Pract* 40:502, 1990.

Hochmeister MN and others: *Effects of Toluidine Blue and destaining reagents used in sexual assault examinations on the ability to obtain DNA profiles from postcoital vaginal swabs.* Paper presented at sexual assault examiner training course, San Diego, June, 1996.

Holmstrom L, Burgess AW: Development of diagnostic categories: sexual traumas, *Am J Nur* 75:1288, 1975.

Hyzer, WG, Krauss TC: The bitemark standard reference scale ABFO No. 2, *J Forens Sci* 33:498, 1988.

Jenny C and others: Sexually transmitted diseases in victims of rape, *N Engl J Med* 322:713, 1990.

Kramer TH and others: Effects of stress on recall, *Appl Cogn Psychol* 5:483, 1991.

Lauber AA, Souma ML: Use of Toluidine Blue for documentation of traumatic intercourse, *Ob Gyn* 60:644, 1982.

Ledray LE: The SANC: A 15 year experience in Minneapolis, *J Emerg Nursing* 18:218, 1992.

Lynch, VA: Forensic nursing: diversity in education and practice, *J Psychosoc Nurs* 31:7, 1993.

McCauley J, Gorman RL, Guzinski G: Toluidine Blue in the detection of perineal lacerations in pediatric and adolescent sexual abuse victims, *Pediatrics* 78:1039, 1986.

McCauley J and others: Toluidine Blue in the corroboration of rape in the adult victim, *Am J Emerg Med* 5:105, 1987.

Minden PB: The victim care services: a program for victims of sexual assault, *Arch Psychiatr Nur* 3:7, 1989.

Mitchell JT: *Personal communication,* March 1996.

Mitchell JT, Everly GS: *Critical incident stress debriefing,* ed 2, Ellicott City, Md, 1996, Chevron.

Norvell MK, Benrubi GI, Thompson RJ: Investigation of microtrauma after sexual intercourse, *J Reprod Med* 29:269, 1984.

Oakleaf L: Rape trauma syndrome, March 1995. Online address: loakleaf@midway.uchicago.edu.

Ochberg FM: Posttraumatic therapy. In Wilson JP, Raphael B, editors: *International handbook of traumatic stress syndromes,* New York, 1993, Plenum Press.

Ochberg FM, editor: *Post-traumatic therapy and victims of violence,* New York, 1988, Brunner/Mazel.

Office of Criminal Justice Planning: *California medical protocol for examination of sexual assault and child sexual abuse victims,* Sacramento, Calif, 1990, the Office.

Pasqualone GA: Forensic RNs as photographers: documentation in the ED, *J Psychosoc Nur* 34:47, 1996.

Rawson RD and others: Analysis of photographic distortion in bitemarks, *J Foren Sci* 31:1262, 1986.

Rimsza, ME: An illustrated guide to adolescent gynecology, *Pediatr Clin North Am* 36:639, 1989.

Secofsky S: *The crime lab.* Paper presented at Sexual Assault Examiner Training Course in Palm Springs, Calif, March 1996.

Seidel HM others: *Mosby's guide to physical examination,* ed 3, St Louis, 1995, Mosby.

Short J and others: Detection of sperm in victim of rape, *N Engl J Med* 424, 1978.

Slaughter L and others: The pattern of genital injury in female sexual assault victims, *Amer J Ob Gyn* 176:609, 1997.

Slaughter L, Brown CRV: Cervical findings in rape victims, *Amer J Ob Gyn* 164:528, 1991.

Slaughter L, Brown CRV: Colposcopy to establish physical findings in rape victims, *Amer J Ob Gyn* 166:83, 1992.

Soules RR and others: The spectrum of alleged rape, *J Reprod Med* 33:1978.

Schwartz MD, Clear TR: Toward a new law on rape, *Crime Delinq* 4:129, 1980.

Smally AJ: Sperm and acid phosphatase examination of the rape patient: medicolegal aspects, *J Fam Pract* 15:170, 1982.

Tanner JM: *Growth at adolescence,* ed 2, Oxford, 1962, Blackwell Scientific.

Thompson WC, Ford S: DNA typing: acceptance and weight of the new genetic identification tests, *Virg Law Rev* 75:45, 1989.

Young WW and others: Sexual assault: review of a National model protocol for forensic and medical evaluation, *Obst & Gyn* 80:878, 1992.

SUGGESTED READINGS

Adams JA, Phillips P, Ahmad M: The usefulness of colposcopic photographs in the evaluation of suspected child sexual abuse, *Adolesc Ped Gyn* 3:75, 1990.

American Board of Forensic Odontology: Guidelines for bite mark analysis, *J Am Dent Assn* 122:383, 1986.

Barber HR: *Geriatric gynecology,* New York, 1988, MacMillan.

Bays J, Lewman LV: Toluidine Blue in the detection at autopsy of perineal and anal lacerations in victims of sexual abuse, *Arch Pathol Lab Med* 116:620, 1992.

Beebe D K: Emergency management of the adult female rape victim, *Am Fam Phys* 43:2041, 1991.

Committee on Infectious Diseases: *Report of the committee on infectious diseases,* ed 22, Elk Grove Village, Ill, 1991, American Academy of Pediatrics.

Fowler JCS and others: Repetitive deoxyribonucleic acid (DNA) and human genome variation-a concise review relevant to forensic biology, *J Foren Sci* 332:1111, 1988.

Goldstein S, Arndt S: *Practice standards for sexual assault nurse examiners.* Paper available through the International Association of Forensic Nurses, 6900 Grove Road; Thorofare, NJ 08086-9447.

Heger A and others: *Evaluation of the sexually abused child,* New York, 1992, Oxford University Press.

Kershner R: Adolescent attitude about rape, *Adolescence* 31: Spring, 1996.

Otto F: *Essential forensic techniques: from rape through examination* (video). (Available from Western Nurse Specialists, 25809-A Business Center Drive, Redlands, CA 92373 [909] 796-6300.)

Silverman EM: Persistence of spermatozoa in the lower genital tracts of women, *J Am Med Assoc* 240:1875. 1978.

Slaughter L, Shackleford S: Genital injury in rape, *Adolesc Ped Gyn* 6:175, 1993.

Wegel JG, Herrin G: Deduction of the order of sexual assaults by DNA analysis of two condoms, *J Foren Sci* 39:844, 1994.

West M: The detection and documentation of trace wound pattern by use of alternative light source, *J Foren Sci* 37:1480, 1992.

Willott GM, Allard, JE: Spermatozoa-their persistence after sexual intercourse, *Foren Sci Intl* 19:135, 1982.

5 ANALYSIS OF CASES

CASES ONE TO FIVE

A. Case Presentation—the Reader

1. Considers the history and laboratory results

2. Identifies the photo findings

3. Concludes whether the findings are consistent with the history and timing of the reported assault

B. Actual Findings and Outcome—the Examiner

1. Identifies actual findings

2. Describes the conclusion to the medical-legal examination

3. Describes the care and treatment

4. Describes the outcome

5. Describes and classifies the perpetrator

Concluding the history and the medical-legal examination, the sexual assault examiner makes a judgment as to whether there has been sexual contact or penetration and if the findings are consistent with the history and timing of the reported assault (Slaughter, Brown, 1991).

The following cases of reported sexual assault provide the reader with an opportunity to consider the history, evaluate the physical injuries on the photographs, and decide whether the photographic findings corroborate the history and timing of the reported assault. The actual findings, outcomes of the cases, and perpetrator types are identified.

1

CASE PRESENTATION

History: A 29-year-old sexually active Caucasian female clerk came to the emergency department 5 hours postassault. She was on a date with a male friend in a hotel room. They were drinking beer and watching cable television. She denied having had consensual intercourse with him. At 5 AM, he awoke and attacked her, restraining her by his weight and with his arms. He forced her legs apart and bruised her legs with the grip of his fingers. While laying supine and on her side, he penetrated her vaginally with his penis and fingers, "two or three times." He unsuccessfully attempted rectal penetration with his penis. He licked her breasts and the left side of her neck, and kissed her lips and breasts, saying, "Tell me you love me." During the examination, she complained of pain in her thighs and head pain.

Laboratories: Rapid plasma reagin (RPR) (nonreactive); *Chlamydia trachomatis* (negative); *Neisseria gonorrhea* (negative); human chorionic gonadotropin (HCG) (negative)

Photographs: On examination, you find the following:

1 External genitalia (Figure 5-1) (×15)

2 External genitalia, after Toluidine Blue dye application and decoloration (Figure 5-2) (×15)

Conclusion: The physical findings (are/are not) consistent with the history and timing of the reported assault.

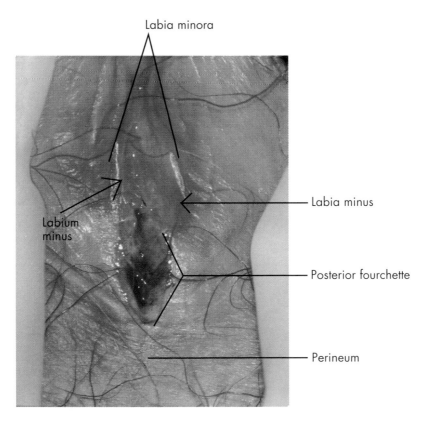

FIGURE 5-1

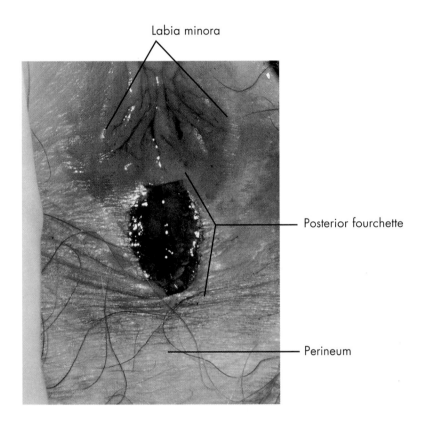

FIGURE 5-2

ACTUAL FINDINGS AND OUTCOME

Findings on Photographs:

1 Laceration of the posterior fourchette; swelling and redness of the labia minora from 3 o'clock to 9 o'clock (Figure 5-3)

2 Distinct Toluidine Blue dye uptake confirming the laceration of the posterior fourchette; dye uptake from 3 o'clock to 9 o'clock on the labia minora indicates an abrasion of the labia minora extending to the posterior fourchette (Figure 5-4)

Actual Conclusion: The findings are consistent with the history and timing of forceful penile vaginal penetration.

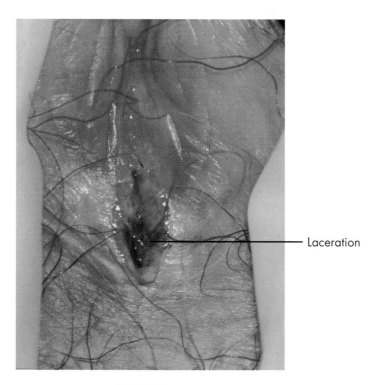

— Laceration

FIGURE 5-3

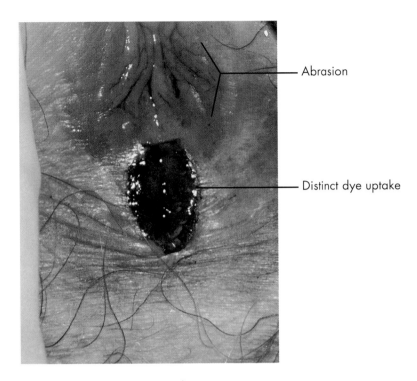

Abrasion

Distinct dye uptake

FIGURE 5-4

Care and Treatment: Teaching was provided as elaborated in Chapter 4, Concluding the Initial Examination, pp. 122–125. Prophylaxis for sexually transmitted diseases (STDs) and pregnancy included the following:

Ceftriaxone (Rocephin) 125 mg, intramuscularly (IM)

Doxycycline (Doxy 100) 100 mg by mouth, twice daily for 7 days

Metronidazole (Flagyl) 500 mg by mouth, twice daily for 7 days

Norgestrel (Ovral) 2 tabs now and 2 tabs in 12 hours

Promethazine (Phenergan) 25 mg by mouth, every 4 to 6 hours as needed for nausea from norgestrel.

She was referred to her health care provider for hepatitis B vaccination (HBV) in three doses at the time of examination, 1 month, and 6 months, as well as for continued care as needed. She was referred to victim advocacy for follow-up counseling.

Outcome: The patient withdrew her testimony before his arrest because she said, "I knew I would never win because I stayed with him the rest of the night."

Perpetrator Classification: Power-reassurance, exploitive, anger, or sadistic; see perpetrator types described in the glossary of this text.

The power-reassurance rapist uses sexual behavior as an expression of rape fantasies. He may believe the victim will actually enjoy it. The assault reassures the perpetrator of his masculinity.

This perpetrator was a 32-year-old, unmarried male janitor who was employed at a fast-food restaurant. He was described by the patient as a "loner." He was a power-reassurance rapist, as evidenced by his surprise attack and minimal aggression. He wanted his victim to show a loving response as evidenced by his licking and kissing, as well as the statement, "Tell me you love me." He took her panties as a souvenir. After the assault, they stayed together until later in the morning. He was trying to make a date with her.

2

CASE PRESENTATION

History: A 22-year-old Hispanic female child care provider came to the emergency department at 9 hours postassault by her husband. The assault began in the kitchen and continued in the living room. She stated he penetrated her vagina at least three times with his penis. She was supine during each penetration. He attempted to penetrate her rectum digitally, and "he stopped when she said it hurt." He forced her to "suck" on his penis by holding her head. He ejaculated in her mouth and on her face. He said she was going to have to "learn to like sex three times a day." During the history, she complained of pain over her genital and anal area.

Laboratories: RPR (nonreactive); *C. trachomatis* (negative); *N. gonorrhea* (negative); HCG (negative)

Photographs: On examination, you find the following:

1 Oral cavity (Figure 5-5) (×15)
2 External genitalia (Figure 5-6) (×15)
3 Perianal area (Figure 5-7) (×15)

Conclusion: The physical findings (are/are not consistent) with the history and timing of the reported assault.

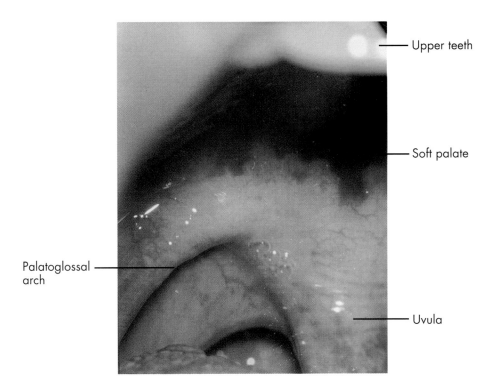

FIGURE 5-5

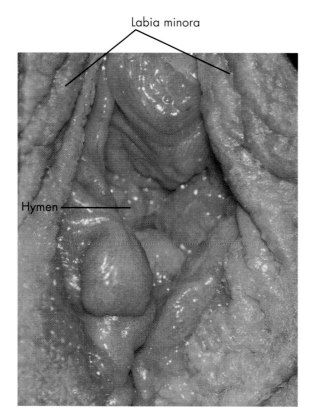

Labia minora

Hymen

FIGURE 5-6

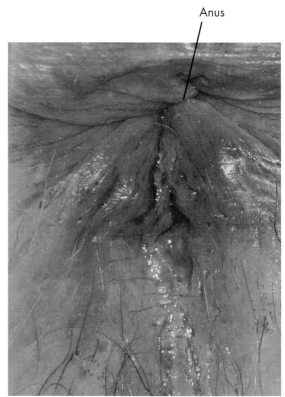

Anus

FIGURE 5-7

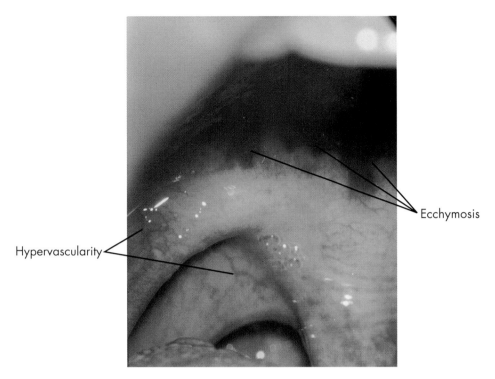

Ecchymosis

Hypervascularity

FIGURE 5-8

ACTUAL FINDINGS AND OUTCOME

Findings on Photographs:

1 Ecchymosis on the soft palate with hypervascularity and focal redness on the uvula and the right arches (Figure 5-8)

2 Generalized redness of the hymen; swelling of the hymen at 11 o'clock to 1 o'clock, and 4 o'clock to 9 o'clock; no lacerations are present (Figure 5-9)

Comparing this photograph with a photograph from the 2-week follow-up examination is critical to clarify the difference between this acute swelling and the normal estrogenized hymen.

3 Redness and swelling around the anus; oozing lacerations and ecchymosis from 5 o'clock to 7 o'clock (Figure 5-10)

Actual Conclusion: Findings are consistent with the history and timing of forceful penile penetration of mouth and vagina. Findings indicate that the anus was also penetrated.

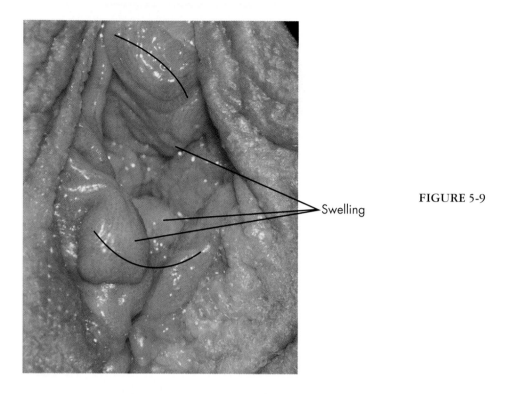

Swelling

FIGURE 5-9

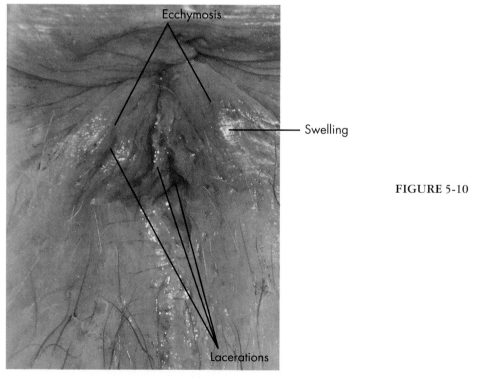

Ecchymosis

Swelling

Lacerations

FIGURE 5-10

Care and Treatment: Teaching was provided as elaborated in Chapter 4, Concluding the Initial Examination, pp. 122–125. Prophylaxis for STDs and pregnancy included the following:

Ceftriaxone (Rocephin) 125 mg IM

Doxycycline, (Doxy 100) 100 mg by mouth, twice daily for 7 days

Metronidazole (Flagyl) 500 mg by mouth, twice daily for 7 days

Norgestrel (Ovral) 2 tabs now and 2 tabs in 12 hours

Promethazine (Phenergan) 25 mg by mouth, every 4 to 6 hours as needed for nausea from norgestrel

She was referred to her health care provider for HBV in three doses at the time of examination, 1 month, and 6 months, as well as for continued care as needed. She was referred to victim advocacy for follow-up counseling.

Outcome: Filing was rejected because prosecution found that her "testimony was not reliable." Furthermore, "spousal cases are difficult to prosecute." At the same time, she withdrew her testimony, stating, "This is my husband."

Perpetrator Classification: Power-reassurance, exploitive, anger, or sadistic; see perpetrator types described in the glossary of this text.

The anger rapist uses sexual behavior as an expression of anger and rage. His intention is to humiliate or punish.

The perpetrator husband, a construction worker, was angry at his wife because she was having intercourse with a mutual friend. He had hit her previously when he was intoxicated. He was intoxicated during this incident, ripped her clothes, used verbal attacks, and threw her onto the bed. He threatened her with future episodes three times per day.

3

CASE PRESENTATION

History: A Caucasian 16-year-old student arrived in the emergency department 20 hours postassault. The assault occurred outside at a Native American reservation. She reported that the stranger, a 30-year-old Mexican male, jumped out from the bushes, hit her in the face, and took off her clothes. While she was lying supine, he forced penile penetration of her vagina twice. She was unsure of ejaculation. He also fondled and kissed her breasts. During the history, she affirmed that she had pain in her right leg and in her back.

Laboratories: RPR (nonreactive); *C. trachomatis* (negative); *N. gonorrhea* (negative); HCG (negative)

Photographs: On examination, you find the following:

   1 External genitalia (Figure 5-11) (×15)

   2 Cervix (Figure 5-12) (×15)

Conclusion: The physical findings (are/are not) consistent with the history and timing of the reported assault.

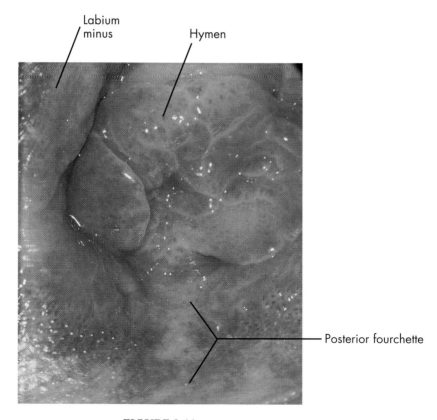

FIGURE 5-11

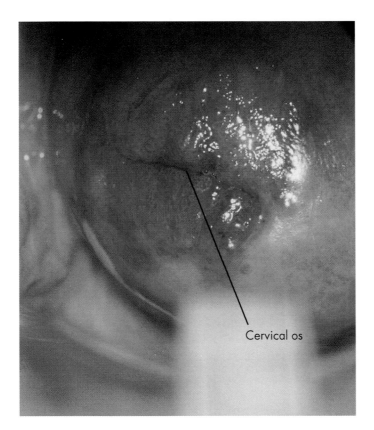

Cervical os

FIGURE 5-12

ACTUAL FINDINGS AND OUTCOME

Findings on Photographs:

1 Generalized blush on all the tissues; hypervascularity of posterior fourchette; no focal redness or TEARS (Figure 5-13)

2 Redness around the cervical os; small amount of clear discharge (Figure 5-14)

An infectious cause for the cervical redness could be determined with cultures, and a follow-up examination is critical to determine if the cervix is typical to this patient.

Actual Conclusion: Physical findings of genitalia are not consistent with the history and timing of forced penile vaginal penetration. The generalized blush of the tissue (see Figure 5-13) is evidence of penile vaginal penetration.

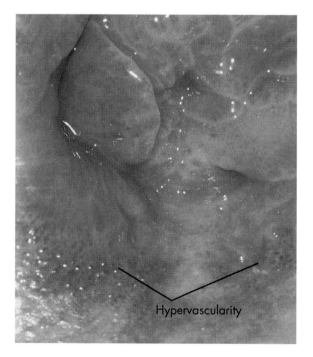

FIGURE 5-13

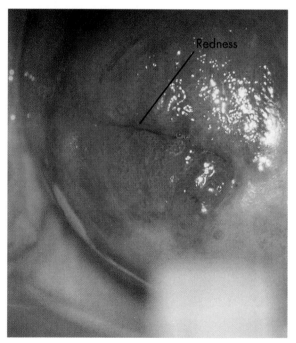

FIGURE 5-14

Care and Treatment: Teaching was provided as elaborated in Chapter 4, Concluding the Initial Examination, pp. 122–125. Prophylaxis for STDs and pregnancy included the following:

Ceftriaxone (Rocephin) 125 mg IM

Doxycycline (Doxy 100) 100 mg by mouth, twice daily for 7 days

Metronidazole (Flagyl) 500 mg by mouth, twice daily for 7 days

Norgestrel (Ovral) 2 tabs now and 2 tabs in 12 hours

Promethazine (Phenergan) 25 mg by mouth, every 4 to 6 hours as needed for nausea from norgesterel

She was referred to her health care provider for HBV in three doses at the time of examination, 1 month, and 6 months, as well as for continued care as needed. She was referred to victim advocacy for follow-up counseling.

Outcome: Several months after this examination, she said that this reported assault was actually consensual intercourse. She reported the rape because her sexual partner was an intravenous (IV) drug user, and she expected to be tested for (human immunodeficiency virus) HIV as part of the medical-legal examination.

Perpetrator Classification: Power-reassurance, exploitive, anger, or sadistic; see perpetrator types described in the glossary.

This was consensual intercourse. False accusation was motivated by the desire for HIV testing.

CASE PRESENTATION

4

History: A 24-year-old single, sexually inactive Hispanic female arrived 2 hours postassault. She reported having been raped by a black male in his mid-twenties who was unknown to the patient. The perpetrator was in the back seat of her unlocked car when she returned from walking. She was forced to drive her car and then stop. He choked her with a rope then pulled her into the backseat on her back. He orally copulated her genitals and rectum. Using his gloved fingers to assist the entry of his flaccid penis, he penetrated her rectum then vagina alternately in two to three cycles. She also felt a cold sharp object enter her vagina and rectum.

He then forced his penis into her mouth. She was forced to manually stimulate the perpetrator's penis while he rubbed her genitals. She was turned to a knee-chest position and he penetrated her vaginally and rectally alternately again in two to three cycles. He ejaculated in her vagina while she was in a knee-chest position. He then dressed, robbed her, and left. The assault duration was estimated at 1 hour, from the patient's abduction to the perpetrator's fleeing. During the history and examination the patient complained of pain in the face, jaw, neck, vagina, rectum, and knees.

Laboratories: RPR (nonreactive); *C. trachomatis* (negative); *N. gonorrhea* (negative); HCG (negative)

Photographs: On examination, you find the following:

1 Neck (Figure 5-15) (35mm)
2 External genitalia (Figure 5-16) (×15)
3 Vaginal wall (Figure 5-17) (×15)
4 Perianal area after Toluidine Blue dye application and decoloration (Figure 5-18) (×15)

Conclusion: The physical findings (are/are not) consistent with the history and timing of the reported assault.

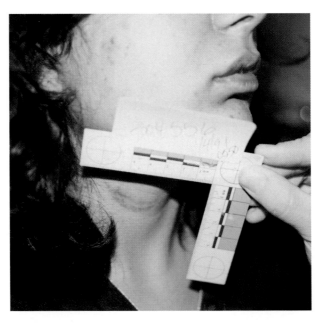

FIGURE 5-15

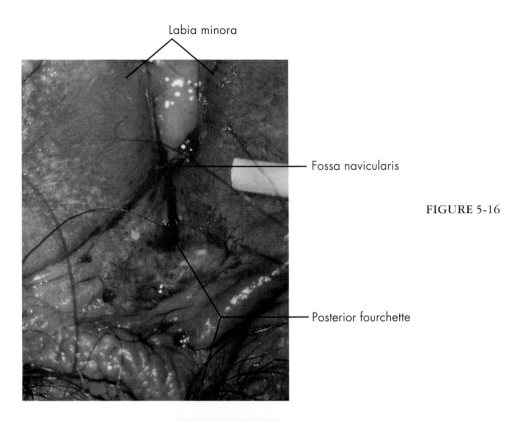

Labia minora

Fossa navicularis

Posterior fourchette

FIGURE 5-16

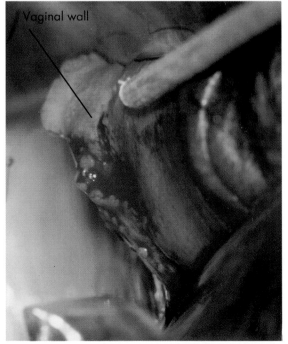

Vaginal wall

FIGURE 5-17

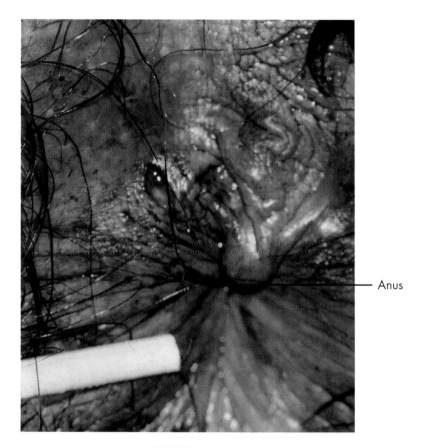

Anus

FIGURE 5-18

ACTUAL FINDINGS AND OUTCOME

Findings on Photographs:

1 Linear abrasions on the right neck 1 cm x 4 cm (Figure 5-19)

2 Swelling and redness of the right and left labia minus and fossa navicularis

   Fresh blood is present from the fossa navicularis, extending to the posterior fourchette. Source of oozing blood is not evident in this photograph (Figure 5-20)

3 Left vaginal wall tear with fresh bleeding (Figure 5-21)

4 Perianal lacerations at 2 o'clock, 10 o'clock, and 11 o'clock (Figure 5-22)

   Toluidine Blue dye is not taken up by these lacerations because of the oozing. The oozing prevents the dye from contacting the nucleated squamous cells in the deeper layers of the epidermis exposed by laceration.

Actual Conclusion: Findings are consistent with the history and timing of forceful digital and penile penetration of the vagina and anus, as well as forceful penile penetration of the mouth.

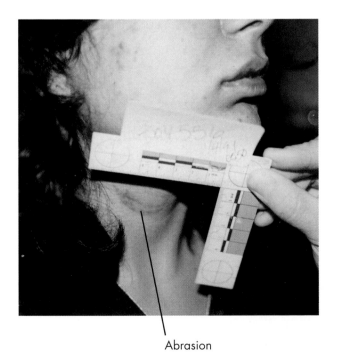

Abrasion

FIGURE 5-19

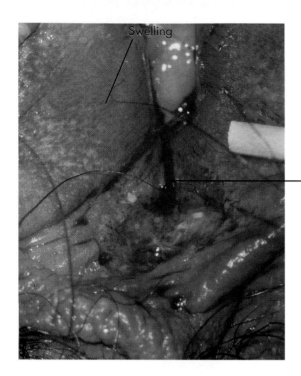

Swelling

Fresh blood ——

FIGURE 5-20

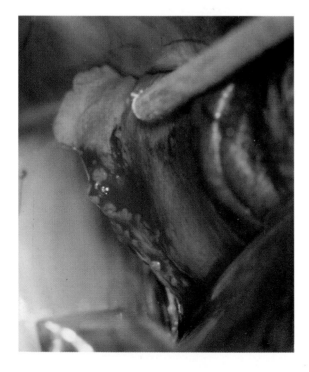

FIGURE 5-21

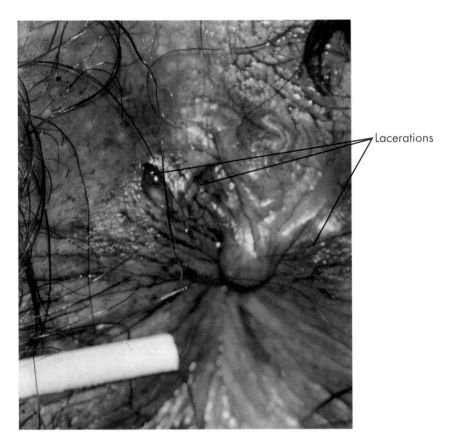

Lacerations

FIGURE 5-22

Care and Treatment: Teaching was provided as elaborated in Chapter 4, Concluding the Initial Examination, pp. 122-125. Prophylaxis for STDs and pregnancy included the following:

Ceftriaxone (Rocephin) 125 mg IM

Doxycycline (Doxy 100) 100 mg by mouth, twice daily for 7 days

Metronidazole (Flagyl) 500 mg by mouth, twice daily for 7 days

Norgestrel (Ovral) 2 tabs now and 2 tabs in 12 hours

Promethazine (Phenergan) 25 mg by mouth, every 4 to 6 hours as needed for nausea from norgestrel

She was referred to her health care provider for HBV in three doses at the time of examination, 1 month, and 6 months, as well as for continued care as needed. She was referred to victim advocacy for follow-up counseling.

Outcome: The perpetrator is at large.

Perpetrator Classification: Power-reassurance, exploitive, anger, or sadistic; see perpetrator types explained in the glossary of this text.

This was an exploitive rapist whose purpose is to express his masculine self-image. He was on the prowl for a woman to exploit sexually as evidenced by him finding an unlocked car and waiting in the car with his ski mask and gloves for the driver's return. He expressed no concern for the victim and punched her face, ripped her clothes, and threatened her several times saying, "I will blow your head off." He had an athletic build and was wearing a sleeveless shirt. She said he smelled of alcohol.

5

CASE PRESENTATION

History: This 21-year-old married, sexually active Caucasian female assembly worker came to the emergency department 7 hours postassault. She was preparing to go to work when her husband pushed her down on the bed, reached into her shorts, and digitally penetrated her vagina. She shouted "no" and tried to push away. He told her to "shut up." He removed her shorts and penetrated her vaginally with his penis. He ejaculated vaginally. Their two toddlers observed the event. She was not taking oral birth control nor other medications.

Laboratories: RPR (nonreactive); *C. trachomatis* (negative); *N. gonorrhea* (negative); HCG (negative)

Photographs: On examination, you find the following:

1 Cervix (Figure 5-23) (×15)

Conclusion: The physical findings (are/are not consistent) with the history and timing of the reported assault.

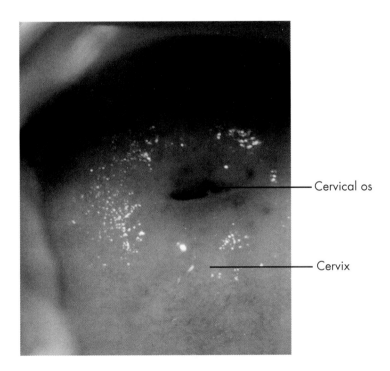

Cervical os

Cervix

FIGURE 5-23

ACTUAL FINDINGS AND OUTCOME

Finding on Photographs:

1 Petechiae around the cervical os from 11 o'clock to 6 o'clock (Figure 5-24)

All other sites were normal. The follow-up examination, conducted at 1 month postassault, revealed the same petechiae pattern around the cervical os.

Actual Conclusion: Findings are not consistent with the history and timing of forceful digital and penile penetration of the vagina.

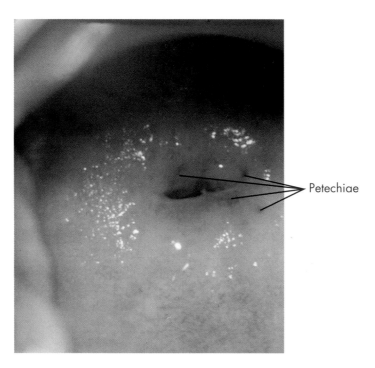

Petechiae

FIGURE 5-24

Care and Treatment: Teaching was provided as elaborated in Chapter 4, Concluding the Initial Examination, pp. 122-125. The following prophylaxis for STDs and pregnancy were offered and accepted:

Ceftriaxone (Rocephin) 125 mg IM

Doxycycline (Doxy 100) 100 mg by mouth, twice daily for 7 days

Metronidazole (Flagyl) 500 mg by mouth, twice daily for 7 days

Norgestrel (Ovral) 2 tabs now and 2 tabs in 12 hours

Promethazine (Phenergan) 25 mg by mouth, every 4 to 6 hours as needed for nausea from norgestrel

She was referred to her health care provider for further evaluation of the cervical petechiae, HBV in three doses at the time of examination, 1 month, and 6 months, as well as for continued care as needed. She was referred to victim advocacy for follow-up counseling.

Outcome: The perpetrator husband plead guilty even though there were minimal findings.

Perpetrator Classification: Power-reassurance, exploitive, anger, or sadistic; see perpetrator types explained in the glossary of this text.

This was an anger rapist. The anger rapist uses sexual behavior as an expression of anger and rage. Their intention is to humiliate or punish. This perpetrator was angry that his wife was having a sexual relationship with another man.

REFERENCE

Slaughter L, Brown RV: Cervical findings in rape victims, *Am J Ob Gyn,* 164:528, 1991.

6 GUIDELINES FOR GIVING EFFECTIVE TESTIMONY

Testifying in a sexual assault case may be stressful, especially if the witness is unexperienced. Witnesses do not choose the line of questioning, nor may they understand the direction of questioning used to clarify a case. They are asked to answer questions using common language in ways that are different from their daily experience in a health care setting. They also may not be allowed to explain their answers. Objections and comments often interrupt the witness' testimony (Freeman, 1992). Furthermore, the witness may face a hostile defendant, a defense attorney whose goal is to discredit the expert witness, and members of a jury who are critical of the expert's opinion. Following guidelines for giving effective testimony as an expert witness helps the witness to be prepared (Arndt, 1995; Freeman, 1992; Montgomery and Thompson, 1996).

GIVING EFFECTIVE TESTIMONY

The task of the expert witness is to present information to help the attorneys, judge, and jury understand specific patient evidence. This is done by providing a qualified, unbiased opinion that is scientifically sound, regarding evidence or a fact (Freeman, 1992). It is not the goal of the professional examiner to offer the opinion that the defendant is guilty or not guilty, nor is it the role of the examiner to act as an advocate for one side or the other. The final decision made by the judge or jury is based on evidence from a comprehensive multidisciplinary investigation, not just the medical-legal examination.

A witness, according to Federal Rule of Civil Procedure 702, is qualified as an expert by knowledge, skill, experience, training, or education (Rodriguez, 1995). Few physicians receive any training in medical school or general residency on the subject of sexual abuse (Heger, Emans, 1992). Therefore nurses and physicians must obtain advanced preparation and continue to practice to be qualified as experts in the care of sexually assaulted patients.

The sexual assault nurse examiner (SANE) is a specialized examiner in the care of sexually assaulted patients (Lenehan, 1991). This specially prepared registered nurse examiner has had at least 80 hours of education and supervised practice in caring for sexually assaulted patients. A SANE is skilled in advanced physical assessment, stabilization of a victim's emotional equilibrium, collection of forensic evidence, and court testimony and procedure (Lynch, 1993). This examiner is a credible expert witness because his or her experience and expertise exceeds that of the generalist emergency department practitioner (Ledray, 1992). Providing care with a specialized examiner is becoming the standard of care.

Although a witness may be an expert in the field, the credibility of that witness is determined by factors other than the educational preparation for the care provided by the examiner. The credibility of a witness is determined by his or her demeanor and character for honesty, the existence of a bias or other motive, and the attitude toward the action in which the witness testified. Also critical to the credibility is the extent of the witness' capacity to communicate, recollect, and perceive. Inconsistent statements or the admission of untruthfulness discredit an expert witness (Otto, 1996).

Preparing to Testify

Evidence

Findings. Review the narrative and photo documentation, organize materials and know the case well before meeting the attorney who is calling you. Be able to substantiate your opinion of whether there is evidence of sexual contact and if the physical findings support the history and timing of the reported incident (Slaughter, Brown, 1991). Keep an inventory of the material reviewed for a specific case (i.e., document, date the document was originated, length of the document, the photographs, and their number and type).

Take photographs of all the injured sites, including comparison sites that were not injured, to the meeting with the attorney. Have normal comparison photos of the injured sites from the patient's follow-up examination or normal findings from other patients. The photographs of normal findings from other patients should show the same Tanner stage and race. Photographs used for comparison should also show the same examination and photographic techniques as the patient's photographs. You should also have comparison photos of sites following consensual intercourse.

After meeting with the attorney who has called you, reorganize the photographs (8″ x 10″ enlargements) or slides of the case according to the attorney's recommendations. Practice and know this set of photographs well enough to describe them without notes. Rehearse your testimony, based on your meeting with the attorney. Avoid presenting it verbatim from practiced sessions.

Expertise

Review your cases, including the number of cases, the age of the patients, and the type of injury they had. Review how many cases you have examined. Update your log each time you are called as a witness. Include the type of witness you were (fact or expert) name of the case, court in which testimony was given, attorney who contacted you, and the outcome. If you have never testified, watch a colleague testify.

Review your goal of presenting the specific and impartial patient evidence. Recall that evidence of bias discredits your testimony. Know the number and types of sexually assaulted patients that are seen at your center per year.

Review your educational preparation; have an updated curriculum vitae prepared. List the special preparation qualifying you as a sexual assault examiner and the content of that preparation. With your list of basic and advanced preparation, indicate your sexual assault–related continuing education, journal subscriptions, relevant association memberships (see Appendix G), articles written, and papers presented on the topic of sexual assault.

Remember you *are* an expert sexual assault examiner, not a generalist. This expertise aids in the identification and documentation of injury and thereby the process of justice. The use of magnification and photodocumentation further supports that expertise. Repeating to oneself phrases such as, "I am knowledgeable, confident, and articulate," helps the examiner project confidence. Examiners that are not experienced or specifically prepared in caring for assault patients may hesitate to record injuries that are not obvious.

Project a professional image by wearing a conservative suit. Appearing relaxed helps to project a demeanor of expertise. Practice relaxation techniques such as deep breathing exercises. If you anticipate seeing your patient outside of court, then ask the advocate to explain to your patient that your presentation as an expert witness includes being cordial but not socializing with them.

Know the steps in the examination. The practice of consistently following a standard protocol for each examination ensures the comprehensiveness and is the most defensible stance in court. Review relevant standards examples, (e.g. the state laws, state Nurse Practice Act, Code of Ethics, and the Standards of Care).

Related Scientific Literature. Review the literature related to the specific injury that has occurred in the case. In addition, review the literature that differentiates findings in consensual versus nonconsensual intercourse. The primary legal issue is not whether intercourse occurred, nor who was the perpetrator, but it is whether that intercourse was consensual. Make enlarged diagrams or models available for further explanation. Know the stages in wound healing.

Prepare a folder containing the initial and follow-up examination documentation, reference material, copies of relevant articles with important sections highlighted. Know the definitions of terms such as penetration, foreign object, rape, and sodomy, which may vary between jurisdictions. Know the spelling of terms such as colposcope and posterior fourchette.

Meet with the attorney contacting you

Be prepared for the question of whether sexual contact or intercourse was consensual or nonconsensual. Remember that the answer to that question is a judiciary judgment. The role of the examiner is to determine whether the findings corroborate the history and timing of the incident and whether there is evidence of sexual contact.

Ask the attorney what is the best way to present an expert opinion, given the strategy and style of the other side. Suggest questions to the attorney that would help order the evidence. Discuss weaknesses or adverse information in the case. Go over new or changed information from the preliminary hearing or trial. Tell the attorney if you have testified before and in what courts. Discuss the cross-examination. Ask the attorney to identify what opposing expert opinion can be expected and responses for questions related to that opposing expert opinion.

If using slides, obtain a slide projector. Bring a laser pointer to court.

Maintain confident, professional, objective, and polite tone and body language. Avoid judgmental statements such as calling the perpetrator names. This detracts from the objectivity of your testimony. Witnesses who come across as an advocate for either side lose credibility. Avoid using humor and be aware of the legal process (Figure 6-1).

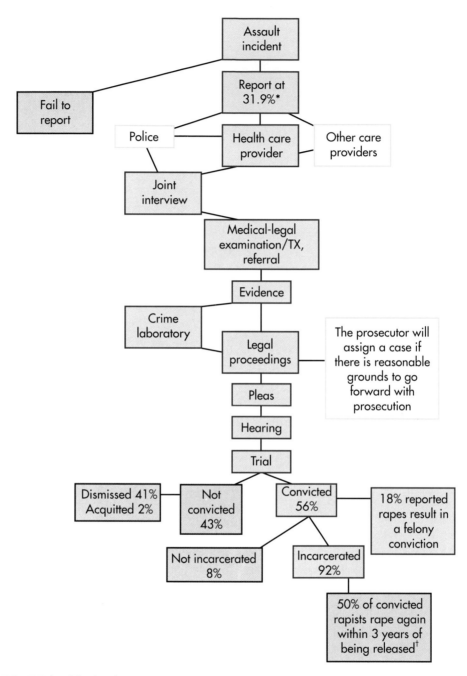

FIGURE 6-1 The legal process.

Adapted from the US Bureau of Justice Statistics, US Department of Justice, Federal Bureau of Investigation, 1993.

[†]*Prodan M: Criminal sexuality. Paper presented at the sexual assault examiner training course, Palm Springs, Calif, March 1995.*

Testifying

General guidelines

Use a confident, polite, and impartial tone and body language. Avoid levity. Anticipate questions according to the meeting you had with the attorney who contacted you. Arrive on time. Write memos or read unrelated reports.

Do not read last-minute material because nothing is "off the record" and anything can be used in court. Do not volunteer information and make no attempt to convince the opposing attorney of the error of his position.

Anticipate the scene as you enter the courtroom. The judge, jurors, and attorneys will all look at you. Look back at them or just over their heads. Anticipate the possibility of hostile body language on the part of the defendant. You will take an oath and answer the first question: "State your name and spell it." Use any relaxation techniques that you have practiced.

Do not socialize with the jurors during breaks. Bring professional journals to read with content unrelated to the case. The jury decides about the believability of a witness and the weight to be given to the testimony based on demeanor and manner of the witness.

Maintain correct posture and face the attorney or jury members to whom you are speaking. Your mind must focus on the question asked and on no one individual's personality, body language, or hostility (Montgomery, Thompson, 1996). When answering the attorney's questions, you may prefer to establish eye contact with one or two people in the jury. Some witnesses prefer to respond to the attorney asking the questions but focus on his or her forehead rather than the eyes.

Speak slowly and loudly enough for the jury across the room to hear you. Think before speaking. Avoid using "nah," "yep," or "I don't know." It is better to say, "I do not recall." Listen to the questions carefully and say, "I don't understand the question," rather than try to answer an unclear question. Do not speculate if you do not know the answer. Be careful about the use of the terms "possibly" and "probably." If you use the term "possibly" it means anything can happen. "Probably" means greater than 50% chance of occurrence (Freeman, 1992). Beware of when the attorney begins a question with, "Is it a fair statement...?" as in, "Is it a fair statement to say this could possibly be accidentally inflicted?" The attorney wants you to agree with him or her, although the concluding part of the statement may be inaccurate or too broad to apply to all cases. Answer the question based on the particular case being litigated. For example, "In this case, that laceration was not accidental."

Clarify which statement or section of an article an attorney is asking about when he or she refers to an article written on a subject. Read the section of the article carefully before responding. Respond only to specific statements or sections in the article because typically, articles have statements with which an examiner may also disagree. Ask the attorney to repeat the question when you are ready to respond.

Both attorneys have formulated a line of questioning, so answer the questions as asked. Do not jump ahead. If an objection is made, stop immediately, even before completing your statement. Do not take offense at objections. Watch for direction from the judge.

Address the judge as "your Honor" and the attorneys as "sir" or "ma'am." At the end of your testimony, you may leave when the judge dismisses you. Avoid waiting in the court after testifying because the jury may wonder about your bias. Furthermore, in some jurisdictions, witnesses are not permitted to observe the trial at which they testify.

Direct examination

Direct examination may require an explanation. Think and organize your answer before responding. Answer each question as asked. The attorney has formulated a line of questions to permit an opinion to be accurately expressed. He or she may ask a central question in various ways. Be consistent about your answer. If you do become aware of an inconsistency, identify the mistake and correct it.

If asked a question such as, "What was your patient like?" ask the judge for permission and quote directly from the documentation. If they ask you if you recognize an item of evidence, respond with "my signature is on the seal of the bag of clothes along with the patient's identification, so those are the pants I obtained and packaged."

Report all the findings as you observed them. Do not try to conform to other witnesses' testimonies or to present part of the facts in an effort to fit what you think is most fair.

As an expert, you are expected to know the scientific literature. Refer to the material you have prepared instead of trying to recall specifics or guessing about the content of that literature.

Cross-examination

The cross examination is an inherent part of the U.S. justice system. The attorneys argue, witnesses present testimony and the jury decides. Techniques of cross examination include suggesting that the expert is biased, dishonest, and uninformed. The cross-examining attorney looks for inconsistencies in the expert's testimony. This side presents a different view of the

expert's testimony through a different line of questioning.

Respond to the defense and prosecution in the same respectful manner. Be confident and if you don't recall, say, "I don't recall." Avoid getting defensive or expressing anger. Avoid obscenity and qualifiers such as, "I guess . . .," or "uh . . . . I think."

Cross-examination usually requires a "yes" or "no" answer. If it is a compound question, answer it in parts. Do not answer a partially untrue question with a "yes" because you may give the incorrect impression of the answer to the second part of the question. If the question is "Was it your opinion that Miss G was vaginally and orally assaulted?" say, "My opinion is that Miss G was vaginally assaulted." The witness may also answer, "There are two parts to that question," and then answer each part.

Answer the questions asked. Do not explain your answer unless you are asked. If the examining attorney just stares at you after you give your answer, by such silence, he or she may be suggesting you continue your explanation. Anticipate this intimidation technique.

If there is any question on how you should proceed, look to the judge for direction. Badgering can be avoided by telling the lawyer that the answer needs to be explained. Anticipate objections from the lawyers and comments from the judge.

Respond to an earlier statement that appears to conflict with another statement by saying, "It is not a contradiction. At the time I believed there to be a bruise there." In the courtroom, truth is the absence of deceit. Do not apologize. If it was an error that you did not mark something on the examination form, say, "Apparently so." Avoid saying, "I guess I should have done that." Avoid statements such as, "That's it," which suggests you have no more to say.

Several days after the proceedings end, speak to the attorney who contacted you. Request recommendations for improving your presentation as a witness. Ask specifically what comments the jury and the defense attorney had about your testimony. Accept these comments for consideration, remembering to maintain the objective perspective of the health care practitioner.

The role of the expert witness as a component in the judicial process is challenging and fulfilling when the witness has prepared the evidence, reviewed his or her qualifications as an expert, and has met with the examining attorney. By following the guidelines for direct and cross-examination, witnesses can present the findings from the medical-legal examination clearly and objectively.

REFERENCES

Arndt S: *Guidelines for being an effective witness.* Paper presented at the sexual assault examiner training course, San Diego, January 1995.

Bureau of Justice Statistics: *Felony defendants in large urban counties, 1990,* NCJ-141872, Washington, DC, 1993, US Department of Justice.

Bureau of Justice Statistics: *National crime victimization survey: victimization levels, preliminary 1995,* Washington DC, 1996, US Department of Justice.

Freeman KR: Testifying as an expert witness. In Heger A, Emans S, editors: *Evaluation of the sexually abused child,* New York, 1992, Oxford University Press.

Heger A, Emans S, editors: *Evaluation of the sexually abused child,* New York, 1992, Oxford University Press.

Ledray LE: The SANC: A 15-year experience in Minneapolis, *J Emerg Nur* 18:218, 1992.

Lenehan GP: Sexual assault nurse examiners: a SANE way to care for rape victims, *J Emerg Nurs* 17:1, 1991.

Lynch VA: Forensic nursing: diversity in education and practice, *J Psychosoc Nurs* 31:10, 1993

Montgomery JT, Thompson D: Surviving the stand: the ED physician as expert witness, *ED Legal Let* 7:21, 1996.

Otto J: *Expert testimony: qualifications of the expert witness.* Paper presented at the sexual assault examiner training course, Palm Springs, Calif, 1996.

Prodan M: *Criminal sexuality.* Paper presented at the sexual assault examiner training course, Palm Springs, Calif, March 1995.

Rodriguez DM: *The expert witness.* Paper presented at Nursing Jurisprudence Workshop, October 5, 1995.

Slaughter L, Brown RV: Cervical findings in rape victims, *Am J Ob Gyn* 164:528, 1991.

SUGGESTED READINGS

Douglas JE, Burgess AW, Burgess AG and others: *Crime classification manual,* New York, 1992, Lexington.

Goldstein S, Arndt S: *Practice standards for sexual assault nurse examiners.* Paper available through the International Association of Forensic Nurses, 6900 Grove Road, Thorofare, NJ 08086-9447.

APPENDICES

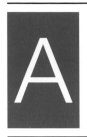

THE MYTHS AND REALITIES OF SEXUAL ASSAULT

VICTIMS

1. *Women respect men for overpowering them. They may even enjoy the rape.*

   In addition to the lack of consent and the coercion and force used, rapists may perform humiliating behaviors like ejaculating into their face, hair, or mouth, urinating or defecating on their victim, forcing anal intercourse, inserting foreign objects into the vagina and rectum or performing anal intercourse followed by oral copulation on the victim.

2. *Only promiscuous and sexually provocative women get raped.*

   There are lifestyles or situations that increase the risk of rape:

   High: Frequenting adult establishments with alcohol use; prostitution; use of drugs; associating with drug users, hitchhikers, or criminals

   Moderate: Car breaks down; individual is physically or mentally disabled

   Victims of sexual assault are from all races, cultures, and ages. However, sexual assault is most prevalent in the 16 to 24-year-old age group and among African Americans (Bureau of Justice Statistics, 1995a). Cases have been reported in which the patients were as young as 15 months and as old as 82 years.

   Testimony regarding the patient's prior sexual history has recently been declared inadmissible as evidence in a court of law in a number of states. The National Commission on the Causes and Prevention of Violence states that discernable victim precipitation of rape occurs in only 4.4% of all cases (Prodan, 1995). This figure is lower than any other violent crimes. However, it is typical for victims to blame themselves for poor choice in selecting friends.

3. *Rape can be avoided by resistance.*

   During the rape the victim may be unable to resist. She may experience shock, fear, and immobility. Her prime motivation is to live. Legally, women no longer have to prove in court that they actively struggled against the rapist.

   Rapes often accompany another crime. The rapist threatens his victim verbally or with fists, a gun, or a knife, and often harms them in nonsexual, as well as sexual, ways. The victim may be beaten, wounded, and sometimes killed. The victim is sometimes referred to as a *survivor* because the victim has lived through the incident. Other times, the term *survivor* is used when the victim has recovered to the point of coping with the incident in a healthy way.

4. *Most rapes are false accusations.*

Estimates indicate that about 10% to 14% of reported rapes are unfounded (Seneski, 1996). In determining an accurate number of sexual assaults, along with the false accusations, the approximately 68% that fail to report must be considered (Bureau of Justice Statistics, 1996).

5. *If a woman stays home, she will be safe from being raped.*

Rape most commonly occurs in a woman's own neighborhood, often inside or near her own home, any time, day or night, and many times, by an acquaintance (Bureau of Justice Statistics, 1995a).

6. *The patient will recover if they just forget about it.*

Most victims develop a pattern of moderate-to-severe rape trauma syndrome (Burgess, Fawcett, Hazelwood and others, 1995). Women report that effects such as shame, humiliation, confusion, fear, and rage last for 1 year or longer, but the memory lasts forever. Many women report symptoms of post-traumatic stress disorder. Some women are able to resume sexual relations with men. Other women become phobic about sexual interactions and have such symptoms as vaginismus (painful spasm of the vagina). The manifestations and the degree of damage depend on the violence of the attack itself, other stressors, precrisis functioning, coping skills, and the support systems she accesses immediately after the attack (Burgess and others, 1995).

MALE VICTIMS

1. *Adult men cannot be raped.*

Men comprise 10% of the sexual assaults treated annually (Bureau, 1995b). It is estimated that assaults of men is nearly that of women, but that only a few men report because of humiliation, lack of support, and unrealistic male sex-role expectations in U.S. society. Homosexual and heterosexual men are most often raped by heterosexual males. Instances where women rape men are extremely rare, as are instances in which homosexual men are the offenders. Male rape occurs not only in institutions, but also in the public sector. Gangs sometimes use male rape to control gang members (Hillman, 1990).

2. *Men become homosexual after being sodomized.*

Gender preference is not communicated through rape. Male rape is legally defined as *sodomy*. Homosexual rape is much more common among men than women, and it often occurs in closed institutions such as prisons and maximum-security hospitals. The crime enables the rapist to discharge aggression and to aggrandize himself. The victim is usually smaller than the rapist, is perceived as passive and "unmanly," and is used as an object. The rapist may be heterosexual, bisexual, or homosexual. The most common act is anal penetration of the victim; the second most common act is oral copulation of the perpetrator (Hillman, 1990).

THE PERPETRATOR

1. *Rapists rape because they "need" sex.*

Most rapes do not occur out of the desire for a sexual partner. Of those who rape, 75% are either married or have regular sexual partners. The three components evident in convicted rapists are power, anger, and sexuality (Groth, Burgess, 1977). There are four different types of rapists (Douglas and others, 1992):

Power rapists: Inadequate men that believe no woman would sleep with them; they are obsessed with fantasies about sex

Exploitive predators: Victimize to gratify their impulses

Anger rapists: Rape is a displaced expression of anger against another person, either female or male

Sexual sadists: Aroused by the pain of their victims

2. *Committing rape represents a momentary lapse in judgment. It is a one-time incident.*

Most rapists commit rape seven times before they are caught. For every "successful" rape, there are 16 to 20 unsuccessful ones (Prodan, 1995). The nationwide rate is increasing—from 1991 to 1992, there was a 1.2% increase per 100,000 people, and from 1983 to 1992, there was a 27% increase (Federal Bureau of Investigation [FBI], 1992). Some of the increase is a result of improved reporting.

3. *Rapists are mentally ill and therefore not responsible for their acts.*

Criminals are responsible for their actions, regardless of what they believe provoked them to commit the crime (Burgess and others, 1995).

4. *Rapists are strangers.*

Most rapes are premeditated. In those incidents against females with lone perpetrators (90% of rapes), 53% are committed by acquaintances, 26% by intimates, 18% by strangers, and 3% by relatives (Bureau of Justice Statistics, 1995a). Ten percent of rapes involve more than one attacker.

Date rape is rape in which the rapist is dating the person he rapes. One college study showed that 38% of male students said that they would commit rape if they thought they could get away with it, 11% said that they had committed rape. In addition, 16% of female students said that they had been raped by men they knew or were dating (Rapaport, Posey 1991).

5. *Most rapes involve black men and white women.*

Of all rapes, 90% are intraracial, 51% involve white perpetrators, 47% involve African American perpetrators who tend to rape African Americans. Two percent are from other races (FBI, 1992).

6. *A man cannot rape his wife.*

Spousal rape is a crime in most U.S. jurisdictions. The idea that a man cannot rape his wife suggests that married women do not have the same right to consent and safety as do single women. Men who force, manipulate, or coerce a spouse into a sex act are committing the crime of rape. Most battered women have experienced some form of sexual abuse in their marriage. It is also known that ex-spouses use rape as a form of retaliation. Spousal rape is rarely reported to law enforcement and when it is reported, it is difficult to prosecute (see Chapter 6).

7. *"My penis is too small to have caused that injury."*

Injury does not correspond to the size of the penis. Erect penis size ranges from 16 to 19 cm in length with an average diameter of 3.5 cm (Masters, Johnson, 1966). Nonconsensual injury occurs where the penis first contacts the perineum. When the patient is supine, it is from 5 o'clock to 7 o'clock on the posterior fourchette, labia minora, hymen, and fossa navicularis (Slaughter, Brown, 1991).

8. *There was no evidence of sperm or acid phosphatase, so there could not have been intercourse.*

In 34% of convicted rapists, sexual dysfunction is apparent: impotence (16%); premature ejaculation (3%); or retarded ejaculation (15%). Only 25% show no sexual dysfunction, whereas, 41% had no data or the assault was resisted or interrupted (Groth, Burgess, 1977). Furthermore, rapists may ejaculate outside the victim or may wear a condom.

9. *If there is no physical injury evident on the patient, rape could not have occurred.*

Conventional protocols for the medical-legal examination have historically yielded positive genital findings in only 10% to 30% of the cases (Cartwright, 1987; Tintinalli, Hoelzer 1985). Colposcopic magnification provides a greater probability of finding injury that is present. There were up to 87% positive findings in patients examined within 48 hours postassault when colposcopic magnification was used during the examination (Slaughter, Brown, 1992). However the medical-legal examination is only one source of evidence to corroborate the sexual assault.

REFERENCES

Bureau of Justice Statistics: *National crime victimization survey: victimization levels, preliminary 1995,* Washington DC, 1996, US Department of Justice.

Bureau of Justice Statistics: *Violence against women: Estimates from the redesigned survey* (NCJ-154348), Washington, DC, 1995a, US Department of Justice.

Bureau of Justice Statistics: *Violent crime* (NCJ-147486), Washington, DC, 1995b, US Department of Justice.

Burgess AW and others: Victim care services and the comprehensive sexual assault assessment tool. In Hazelwood RR and Burgess AW, editors: *Practical aspects of rape investigation,* Boca Raton, Fla, 1995, CRC Press.

Cartwright PS: Factors that correlate with injury sustained by survivors of sexual assault, *Ob Gyn* 70:44, 1987.

Douglas JE and others: *Crime classification manual,* New York, 1992, MacMillan.

Federal Bureau of Investigation: Crimes and crime rates, by type: 1983 to 1992, *Crime in the United States,* No 301, 1992, the Bureau.

Groth AN, Burgess AW: Sexual dysfunction during rape, *N Eng J Med* 297:764, 1977.

Hickson GCI and others: Gay men as victims of nonconsensual sex, *Arch Sex Behav* 23:281, 1994.

Hillman R: Male victims of sexual assault, *Brit J Gen Pract* 40:502, 1990.

Masters WH and Johnson VE: *The human sexual response,* Boston, 1966, Little Brown.

Prodan M: *Criminal sexuality.* Paper presented in Palm Springs, Calif, March 1995.

Rapaport KR, Posey CD: Sexually coercive college males. In Parrot A, editor: *Acquaintance rape: the hidden crime,* New York, 1991, John Wiley & Sons.

Seneski PC: *False allegations of sexual assault.* Paper presented in Palm Springs, Calif, March 1996.

Slaughter L, Brown C: Colposcopy to establish physician findings in rape victims, *Am J Obstet Gynecol* 166:83, 1992.

Tintinalli JE, Hoelzer M: Clinical findings and legal resolution in sexual assault, *Ann Emerg Med* 14:447, 1985.

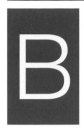
B RESOURCES FOR PATIENT SELF-HELP

SUPPORT PROGRAMS

National Adolescent Perpetrator Network
(303) 321-3963

National Children's Advocacy Center
Information for adolescents and children; local sites offer therapy for patients and training for professionals; (205) 533-KIDS; **e-mail:** ncac@hiwaay.net

National Coalition Against Sexual Assault
Individuals and networks of rape crisis centers and related agencies working against sexual assault through education, public policy advocacy, and coalition building; 125 North Enola Drive, Enola, PA 17025; (717) 728-9740, FAX (717) 728-9781; **e-mail:** ncasa@redrose.net; URL: www.achiever.com/freehmpg.ncas

National Committee to Prevent Child Abuse
Provides public information concerning the abuse of children and adolescents; (800) 835-2671 or (312) 663-3520

National Hospital for Kids in Crisis
An acute care psychiatric hospital dedicated to children and adolescents experiencing life-threatening crises, depression, and family crisis; (800) 44-MY-KID

National Organization for Victim Assistance
Dedicated to professional development through education and training, a voice in state legislatures, and membership communication, as well as to victims by providing 24-hour crisis counseling and follow-up assistance; 1757 Park Road NW Washington, DC 20010; (202) 232-6682 or (800) TRY-NOVA

National Victim's Constitutional Amendment Network
URL: www.ncv.org/nvcan

National Victims' Center
Provides information, counseling, and referral to victims; (800) FYI-CALL, FAX: (212) 753-0149

National Women's Studies Association
Referral to local colleges that have women's studies programs or courses; 7100 Baltimore Avenue, Suite 301, University of Maryland, College Park, MD 20740; (301) 403-0524

Office for Victims of Crime Resource Center
To access reports from the National Criminal Justice Office; (800) 627-6872

Rape: Abuse and Incest National Network
Offers no-cost crisis intervention and counseling; call for local office; (800) 656-4673

Red Flag/Green Flag Resources
Provides sexual abuse prevention materials for children and young women; (800) 627-3675; **e-mail:** rfgf@netcenter.net URL:www.redflag-green.com

Survivor Connections

Network and referral by clergy, family, youth leaders, counselors, and others specifically for survivors of sexual assault; 52 Lyndon Road, Cranston, RI 02905-1121; (401) 941-2548

SELF-DEFENSE AND PERSONAL EMPOWERMENT

To be skilled at the martial arts takes years of preparation and practice. Various other programs are designed to help with personal safety:

Defensive Awareness Training Academy

229 East Evergreen, Redmond, OR 97756; (888) BE-SAFE

Model Mugging of San Luis Obispo

P.O. Box 986, San Luis Obispo, CA 93406

Personal Empowerment and Model Mugging

(800) 77FIGHT or (212) 650-9546

Additional self-defense classes may be found through the local telephone directory under key words such as *schools* or *self-defense*, or by contacting the local rape crisis center for a referral.

BOOKS

This is an alphabetical-by-author list of sample books. Check the self-help section of your local bookstore for additional readings. Read the preface or back cover to determine what best meets your needs.

Brownmiller S: *Against our will: men, women, and rape,* New York, 1975, Simon & Schuster.

Carosella, C, editor: *Who's afraid of the dark?* New York, 1995, HarperCollins.

Fairstein L: *Sexual violence: our war against rape,* New York, 1993, William Morrow.

Koss M: *The rape victim,* Newberry Park, Calif, 1991, Sage.

Maltz W: *The sexual healing journey,* New York, 1991, HarperCollins.

Tesoro M: *Options for avoiding assault: a guide to assertiveness, boundaries, and de-escalation for violent confrontation,* San Luis Obispo, Calif, 1994, SDEN Publications (Box 986, San Luis Obispo, CA 93406).

Tuttle C: *The path to wholeness,* American Fork, UT, 1995, Covenant Communications.

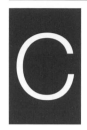

C FOLLOW-UP CARE INSTRUCTIONS: A MODEL

REFERRALS

Private Physician_____ OB/Gyn_____

_____ _____

Counseling

EYE Counseling and
   Crisis Service
200 N. Ash, Suite 110
Escondido, CA 92027
(619) 747-6281

Women's Resource
   Center
3355 Mission Avenue
  #110
Oceanside, CA 92054
(619) 757-3500

1. *Evidence*

   You have been examined and specimens have been obtained for law enforcement to be used as evidence. We have also done a test to determine whether you are pregnant. We need the information to determine if we can offer you a medication to prevent pregnancy.

2. *Follow-up instructions*

   - See a physician in 10 to 14 days to test for successful prevention of gonorrhea and chlamydia and to begin hepatitis B vaccine (HBV) series: *first of 3 doses at time of examination, at 1 month, and at 6 months.* The use of hepatitis B immune globulin (HBIG) combined with vaccination can prevent infection among persons exposed sexually to HBV if administered within 14 days of exposure (CDC, 1993). Ask about and plan for human immunodeficiency virus (HIV) testing.

   - See a physician in 4 to 6 weeks for a syphilis test and repeat pregnancy test if needed.

   - See a counselor to help in dealing with this experience. Listed at left are two counseling centers, but others are available. Ask specifically for a counselor experienced with sexually assaulted persons.

   - Call the sexual assault office here if you have other questions: (619) 485-4455

3. *Medications*

   You have been given the following medications:

   FOR SEXUALLY TRANSMITTED DISEASE (CDC, 1993):

   - *Gonorrhea:* Ceftriazone 125 mg IM in a single dose
   - *Chlamydia:* Doxycycline 100 mg by mouth two times daily for 7 days or tetracycline hydrochloride 500 mg by mouth 4 times daily for 7 days
   - *Trichomoniasis and bacterial vaginosis:* Metronidazole 2 gm by mouth in a single dose.

   Take each medication as directed, until it is gone. Abstain from sexual intercourse until medications are completed.

TO PREVENT PREGNANCY:

If the pregnancy test was negative, you are offered norgestrel (Ovral), 2 tabs (100 mcg ethinyl estradiol) at the time of the examination and 2 tabs in 12 hours with promethazine (Phenergan) 25 mg by mouth every 4 to 6 hours as needed for nausea.

OTHER:

- Tetanus 0.5 ml IM now if last tetanus was greater than 5 years ago

Lot #: _____ Exp. date: _____
Manufacturer: _____

- Acetaminophen 1 gm by mouth as needed in a single dose, for discomfort

4. *Follow-up examination:*

Return here on (date): _____ and (time): _____ for your follow-up examination to evaluate your healing and response to the medications.

D HIGHLIGHTS OF THE MEDICAL-LEGAL EXAMINATION

The following criteria aid in the medical-legal examination of a patient within 72 hours postassault:

1. *Identification:* Patient, examiner
2. *Explanation:* Setting, consents history and examination, photographs
3. *Initial evidence*
   A. ORAL: Two swabs, two dry mounts, saliva sample, gonorrhea, chlamydia culture per protocol and history
   B. BLOOD: Syphilis serology, pregnancy, crime laboratory serology and alcohol
   C. URINE: For toxicology and pregnancy; if patient wipes, collect tissue
4. *History*
   A. Chronology of assault, place, position, actions subsequent to the assault
   B. General medical history (last menstrual period, parity, last intercourse, loss of consciousness, medications, no known allergies)
   C. Perpetrator (sexual dysfunction, alcohol use, unique features)
5. *Physical examination:* Document and photograph (35mm and magnified views)
   A. GENERAL APPEARANCE: Affect, vital signs, height, weight, allergies, medications
   B. CLOTHING: Appearance, Wood's Lamp, collect secretions, collect clothes without shaking
   C. GENERAL BODY EXAMINATION: Visual for TEARS*, bite marks, scan with Wood's Lamp, collect secretions and debris
      1. Head (cut matted hair, reference samples from head, body, face [males])
      2. Fingernails (scrapings; cut and collect broken edges)
      3. Lips and mouth
   D. EXTERNAL GENITALIA: For TEARS, scan with Wood's Lamp and collect secretions and debris; cut matted pubic hair, then comb for debris
      Males (2 penile swabs (glans/shaft); per protocol, urethral swab for gonorrhea and chlamydia)
   E. VAGINA AND CERVIX: For TEARS, collect two shallow and two deep swabs: prepare two dry mounts and one wet mount. Immediately check the wet mount for sperm. Collect one cervical swab. Endocervical culture for gonor-

*T: tear (laceration); E: ecchymosis (bruise); A: abrasion; R: redness (erythema); S: swelling (edema)

173

rhea and chlamydia per protocol

F. ANUS: For TEARS, collect secretions and debris, collect two anal swabs, prepare two dry mounts. Perform anoscopy and check for TEARS. Collect gonorrhea and chlamydia culture per protocol

6. *Care of Evidence*

   A. PRINCIPLES

   1. Cool air dry all specimens for 1 hour

   2. Label all containers (name of patient, date, contents, location on body where taken or from what swab mount was made, collection site, initials of collector)

   B. HOSPITAL LABORATORY

   1. Cultures for gonorrhea and chlamydia (oropharynx, cervical, anal, urethral)

   2. Pregnancy (blood or urine)

   C. CRIME LABORATORY

   1. Blood specimens (blood typing, rapid plasma reagin, hepatitis, toxicology, HIV test per protocol)

   2. Clothing in separate paper bags

   3. General body (debris and dried secretions on clothing and body)

   4. Fingernail scrapings

   5. Oral (two swabs from oral cavity and two dry mounts)

   6. Genitalia (dried secretion, debris, matted hair, combings; penile swabs)

   7. Vaginal/cervical (four swabs, one wet, two dry mounts, and washing)

   8. Anal (two swabs, two dry mounts, dried secretions and debris)

7. *Document*

   1. Evidence collected, including rolls of film, video

   2. Findings consistent/inconsistent with history and time frame given by the patient

   3. Evidence of sexual intercourse

8. *Conclude With Patient*

   1. Teach (findings, medications, follow-up, emotional care, prevention handouts)

   2. Treat (antibiotics, emergency contraceptive [if negative pregnancy test])

   3. Connect (to victim advocacy services, rape crisis numbers)

   4. Check (organize evidence, check labels, distribute and secure evidence)

9. *Follow-up Examination*

   1. Examine

   2. Teach

   3. Connect

   4. Check

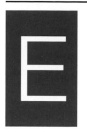

THE MEDICAL REPORT FOR SUSPECTED ACUTE ADULT/ADOLESCENT SEXUAL ASSAULT (OCJP 923)*

As of May 1997, a revised OCJP 923 and guidelines are in development (the format will be changed and additions such as these will be made).

HISTORY

- Last consenting intercourse: Intravaginal ejaculation? Type of condom used?
- Parity, gravidity
- Drugs and/or alcohol used within the last 12 hours of assault?
- Ate or drank what since assault?
- Douched? With what?
- Injuries to the perpetrator? Describe.

METHODS EMPLOYED BY THE PERPETRATOR

- Forced/coerced the use of drugs or alcohol?
- Condom used? Type? Location?
- Penis circumsized?

PHOTODOCUMENTATION

- Parts photographed
- Type photography used

FINAL ASSESSMENT

- A new category—*Interpretation pending consultation*

NOTE: The form OCJP 925 is used for child or adolescent under 14 years.

---

*Office of Criminal Justice Planning (OCJP) Form 923, State of California

State of California   Office of Criminal Justice Planning (OCJP) 923

MEDICAL REPORT—SUSPECTED SEXUAL ASSAULT

Patients requesting examination, treatment and evidence collection: Penal Code § 13823.5 requires every physician who conducts a medical examination for evidence of a sexual assault to use this form to record findings. Complete each part of the form and if an item is inapplicable, write N/A.

Patients requesting examination and treatment only: Penal Code § 11160–11161 requires physicians and hospitals to notify a law enforcement agency by telephone and in writing if treatment is sought for injuries inflicted in violation of any state penal law. If the patient consents to treatment only, complete Part A # 1 and 2, Part B # 1, and Part E # 1–10 to the extent it is relevant to treatment, and mail this form to the local law enforcement agency.

Minors: Civil Code § 34.9 permits minors, 12 years of age or older, to consent to medical examination, treatment, and evidence collection related to a sexual assault without parental consent. Physicians are required, however, to attempt to contact the parent or legal guardian and note in the treatment record the date and time the attempted contact was made including whether the attempt was successful or unsuccessful. This provision is not applicable if the physician reasonably believes the parent or guardian committed the sexual assault on the minor. If applicable, check here ( ) and note the date and time the attempt to contact parents was made in the treatment record.

Liability and release of information: No civil or criminal liability attaches to filling out this form. Confidentiality is not breached by releasing it to law enforcement agencies.

A. GENERAL INFORMATION
(print or type)   Name of Hospital:

1. Name of patient					Patient ID number			

2. Address		City		County	State	Phone (W) (H)	

3. Age	DOB	Sex	Race	Date/time of arrival	Date/time of exam	Date/time of discharge	Mode of transportation

4. Phone report made to law enforcement agency: Name of officer	Agency		ID number	Phone

5. Responding officer	Agency		ID number	Phone

B. PATIENT CONSENT

1. I understand that hospitals and physicians are required by Penal Code § 11160–11161 to report to law enforcement authorities cases in which medical care is sought when injuries have been inflicted upon any person in violation of any state penal law. The report must state the name of the injured person, current whereabouts, and the type and extent of injuries.

                                            Patient/Parent/Guardian (circle)

2. I understand that a separate medical examination for evidence of sexual assault at public expense can, with my consent, be conducted by a physician to discover and preserve evidence of the assault. If conducted, the report of the examination and any evidence obtained will be released to law enforcement authorities. I understand that the examination may include the collection of reference specimens at the time of the examination or at a later date. Knowing this, I consent to a medical examination for evidence of sexual assault. I understand that I may withdraw consent at any time for any portion of the evidential examination.

                                            Patient/Parent/Guardian (circle)

3. I understand that collection of evidence may include photographing injuries and that these photographs may include the genital area. Knowing this, I consent to having photographs taken.

                                            Patient/Parent/Guardian (circle)

4. I have been informed that victims of crime are eligible to submit crime victim compensation claims to the State Board of Control for out-of-pocket medical expenses, loss of wages, and job retraining and rehabilitation. I further understand that counseling is also a reimbursable expense.

                                            Patient/Parent/Guardian (circle)

C. AUTHORIZATION FOR EVIDENTIAL EXAM

I request a medical examination and collection of evidence for suspected sexual assault of the patient at public expense.

                                 Law Enforcement Officer

                                 Agency   ID Number   Date

DISTRIBUTION OF OCJP 923 FOR EVIDENTIAL EXAMS ONLY	HOSPITAL IDENTIFICATION INFORMATION
ORIGINAL TO LAW ENFORCEMENT; PINK COPY TO CRIME LAB (SUBMIT WITH EVIDENCE); YELLOW COPY TO HOSPITAL RECORDS	

OCJP 923   86 96699

FIGURE E-1   The OCJP 923 form.

D. OBTAIN PATIENT HISTORY. RECORDER SHOULD ALLOW PATIENT OR OTHER PERSON PROVIDING HISTORY TO DESCRIBE INCIDENT(S) TO THE EXTENT POSSIBLE AND RECORD THE ACTS DESCRIBED BELOW. DETERMINE AND USE TERMS FAMILIAR TO THE PATIENT. FOLLOW-UP QUESTIONS MAY BE NECESSARY TO ENSURE THAT ALL ITEMS ARE COVERED.

1. Name of person providing history	Relationship to patient	Date/time of assault(s)

2. Location and physical surroundings of assault (bed, field, car, rug, floor, etc.)

3. Name(s), number and race of assailant(s)

4. Acts described by patient
(Any penetration, however slight, of the labia or rectum by the penis or any penetration of a genital or anal opening by a foreign object or body part constitutes the act. Oral copulation and masturbation only require contact.)

	Yes	No	Attempted	Unsure	If more than one assailant, identify person.
Penetration of vagina by					
Penis					
Finger					
Foreign object					
Describe the object					
Penetration of rectum by					
Penis					
Finger					
Foreign object					
Describe the object					
Oral copulation of genitals					
of victim by assailant					
of assailant by victim					
Oral copulation of anus					
of victim by assailant					
of assailant by victim					
Masturbation					
of victim by assailant					
of assailant by victim					
other					

Did ejaculation occur
outside a body orifice?
if yes, describe the location
on the body.
Foam, jelly, or condom used
(circle)

Lubricant used

Fondling, licking or kissing
(circle)
If yes, describe the location
on the body.
Other acts

5. Physical injuries and/or pain described by patient

	Yes	No
Lapse of consciousness:		
Vomited:		
Pre-existing physical injuries:		

If yes, describe: _____

8. Pertinent medical history

Last menstrual period:

Any recent (60 days) anal-genital injuries, surgeries, diagnostic procedures, or medical treatment which may affect physical findings? ( ) Yes ( ) No

If yes, record information in separate medical chart.

Consenting intercourse within past 72 hours? ( ) Yes ( ) No

Approximate date/time:

DO NOT RECORD ANY OTHER INFORMATION REGARDING SEXUAL HISTORY ON THIS FORM.

6. Methods employed by perpetrator

	Yes	No	Area of body
Weapon inflicted injuries			
Type of weapon(s)			
Physical blows by hands or feet (circle)			
Grabbing/grasping/holding (circle)			
Physical restraints Type(s) used			
Bites			
Choking			
Burns (including chemical/toxic)			
Threat(s) of harm			

To whom:
Type of threat(s)
Other method(s) used
Describe:

7. Post-assault hygiene/activity
( ) Not applicable if over 72 hours

	Yes	No
Urinated		
Defecated		
Genital wipe/wash		
Bath/shower		
Douche		
Removed/inserted tampon, sponge, diaphragm (circle)		
Brushed teeth		
Oral gargle/swish		
Changed clothing		

HOSPITAL IDENTIFICATION INFORMATION

OCJP 923

86 96699

FIGURE E-1—cont'd   The OCJP 923 form.

E. CONDUCT A GENERAL PHYSICAL EXAM AND RECORD FINDINGS. COLLECT AND PRESERVE EVIDENCE FOR EVIDENTIAL EXAM

1. Blood pressure	Pulse	Temperature	Respiration	2. Height	Weight	Eye color	Hair color

3. Note condition of clothing upon arrival (rips, tears, presence of foreign materials)

4. Collect outer and underclothing worn during or immediately after assault.

5. Collect fingernail scrapings, if indicated.

6. Record general physical appearance:

- Record injuries and findings on diagrams: erythema, abrasions, bruises (detail shape), contusions, induration, lacerations, fractures, bites, burns, and stains/foreign materials on the body.
- Record size and appearance of injuries. Note swelling and areas of tenderness.
- Collect dried and moist secretions, stains, and foreign materials from the body including the head, hair, and scalp. Identify location on diagrams.
- Scan the entire body with a Wood's Lamp. Swab each suspicious substance or fluorescent area with a separate swab. Label Wood's Lamp findings "W.L."
- Collect the following reference samples at the time of the exam if required by crime lab: saliva, head, hair, and body/facial hair from males.
- Record specimens collected on Section 11.

7. Examine the oral cavity for injury and the area around the mouth for seminal fluid. Note frenulum trauma.

- If indicated by history: Swab the area around the mouth. Collect 2 swabs from the oral cavity up to 6 hours post-assault for seminal fluid. Prepare two dry mount slides.
- If indicated by history, take a GC culture from the oropharynx and offer prophylaxis. Take other STD cultures as indicated.
- Record specimens collected on Section 11.

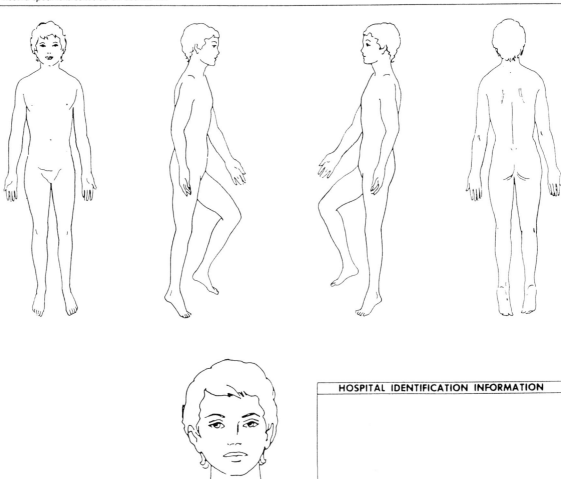

OCJP 923

86 96699

HOSPITAL IDENTIFICATION INFORMATION

FIGURE E-1—cont'd   The OCJP 923 form.

8. External genitalia
- Examine the external genitalia and perianal area including the inner thighs for injury and foreign materials.
- Collect dried and moist secretions and foreign materials. Identify location on diagrams.
- Cut matted pubic hair. Comb pubic hair to collect foreign materials.
- Scan area with Wood's Lamp. Swab each suspicious substance or fluorescent area. Label Wood's Lamp findings "W.L."
- Collect pubic hair reference samples at time of exam if required by crime lab.
- For males, collect 2 penile swabs if indicated. Collect one swab from the urethral meatus and one swab from the glans and shaft. If indicated by history, take a GC culture from the urethra and offer prophylaxis. Take other STD cultures as indicated.
- Record specimens collected on Section 11.

9. Vagina and cervix
- Examine for injury and foreign materials.
- Collect 3 swabs from vaginal pool. Prepare 1 wet mount and 2 dry mount slides. Examine wet mount for sperm. Take a GC culture from the endocervix and offer prophylaxis. Take other STD cultures as indicated.
- If the assault occurred more than 24 hours prior to the exam, collection of cervical swabs may be indicated up to 2 weeks post-assault if no possibility exists of contaminating the specimen with semen from previous coitus. Label cervical swabs and slides to distinguish them from the vaginal swabs and slides.
- Aspirate/washings to detect sperm are optional.
- Record specimens collected on Section 11.
- Obtain pregnancy test (blood or urine).

10. Anus and rectum
- Examine the buttocks, perianal skin, and anal folds for injury.
- Collect dried and moist secretions and foreign materials. Foreign materials may include lubricants and fecal matter.
- If indicated by history and/or findings: Collect 2 rectal swabs and prepare 2 dry mount slides. Avoid contaminating rectal swabs by cleaning the perianal area and dilating the anus using an anal speculum.
- Conduct an anoscopic or proctoscopic exam if rectal injury is suspected.
- If indicated by history, take a GC culture from the rectum and offer prophylaxis. Take other STD cultures as indicated.
- Record specimens collected on Section 11.
- Take blood for syphilis serology. Offer prophylaxis.

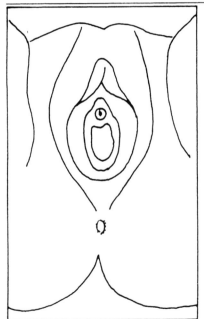 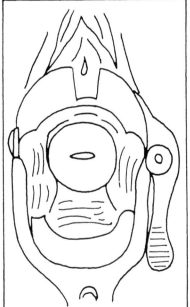 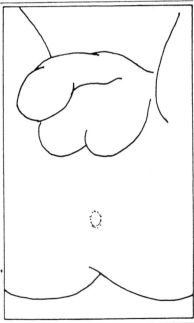

HOSPITAL IDENTIFICATION INFORMATION

OCJP 923   86 96699

FIGURE E-1—cont'd   The OCJP 923 form.

11. Record evidence and specimens collected.

ALL SWABS AND SLIDES MUST BE AIR DRIED PRIOR TO PACKAGING (PENAL CODE § 13823.11). AIR DRY UNDER A STREAM OF COOL AIR FOR 60 MINUTES. Swabs and slides must be individually labeled, coded to show which slides were prepared from which swabs, and time taken. All containers (tubes, bindles, envelopes) for individual items must be labeled with the name of the patient, contents, location of the body where taken, and name of hospital. Package small containers in a large envelope and record chain of custody. See the State of California Medical Protocol for Examination of Sexual Assault and Child Sexual Abuse Victims published by the state Office of Criminal Justice Planning, 1130 K Street, Sacramento, CA 95814 (916) 324-9100 for additional information.

SPECIMENS FOR PRESENCE OF SEMEN, SPERM MOTILITY, AND TYPING TO CRIME LAB

	Swabs	Dry mount slides	Yes	No	N/A	Taken by	Time
Oral							
Vaginal							
Rectal							
Penile							
Aspirate/washings (optional)							

Vaginal wet mount slide examined for spermatozoa, dried, and submitted to crime lab					
Motile sperm observed					
Non-motile sperm observed					

OTHER EVIDENCE TO CRIME LAB

	Yes	No	N/A	Taken by
Clothing				
Fingernail Scrapings				
Foreign materials on body				
Blood				
Dried secretions				
Fiber/loose hair				
Vegetation				
Dirt/gravel/glass				
Matted pubic hair cuttings				
Pubic hair combings				
Comb				
Swabs of bite marks				
Control swabs				
Photographs				
Area of the body _____				
Type of camera _____				
Other _____				

_____
_____
_____

REFERENCE SAMPLES AND TOXICOLOGY SCREENS TO CRIME LAB

Reference samples and toxicology screens can only be collected with the consent of the patient. Reference samples can be collected at the time of the exam or at a later date according to crime lab policies. Toxicology screens should be collected at the time of the exam upon the recommendation of the physical examiner or law enforcement officer.

Reference samples

	Yes	No	N/A	Taken by
Blood typing (yellow top tube)				
Saliva				
Head hair				
Pubic hair				
Facial/body hair				

Toxicology screens

Blood/alcohol toxicology (grey top tube)				
Urine toxicology				

EXAM INFORMATION (print)

Anoscopic exam			
Proctoscopic exam			
Genital exam done with:			
Direct visualization			
Colposcope			
Hand held magnifier			

PERSONNEL INVOLVED (print)	PHONE
History taken by:	
Physical examination performed by:	
Specimens labeled and sealed by:	
Assisting nurse:	

FINDINGS

Report of sexual assault, exam reveals:

☐ PHYSICAL FINDINGS   ☐ NO PHYSICAL FINDINGS
   ☐ Exam consistent with history   ☐ Exam consistent with history
   ☐ Exam inconsistent with history   ☐ Exam inconsistent with history

SUMMARY OF FINDINGS

PHYSICAL EXAMINER

Print name of physical examiner

Signature of physical examiner

License number of physical examiner

LAW ENFORCEMENT OFFICER

I have received the indicated items as evidence and the original of this report.

Law enforcement officer

Law enforcement agency   ID number   Date

HOSPITAL IDENTIFICATION INFORMATION

ARRANGE FOLLOW-UP FOR STD, PREGNANCY, INJURIES, AND PROVIDE REFERRALS FOR PSYCHOLOGICAL CARE.

OCJP 923   86 96699

FIGURE E-1—cont'd   The OCJP 923 form.

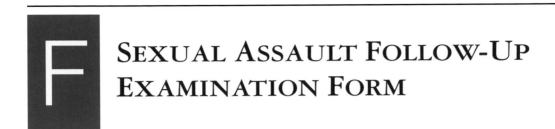

F SEXUAL ASSAULT FOLLOW-UP EXAMINATION FORM

4/96

**PPHS
Follow-Up Examination (SART)
Face Sheet**

Patient Name _____ MR#: _____

Date of initial forensic examination: _____

Date of follow-up examination: _____

Problems since initial examination: _____

_____

_____

_____

_____

_____

No Show: _____ Attempts to Contact: _____

Comments:_____

_____

_____

_____

_____

SART FOLLOW-UP EXAMINATION

TODAY'S DATE _____   **DATE INITIAL SART EXAMINATION** _____   **INTERVAL** _____

BIRTH CONTROL METHOD _____

	YES	NO	DESCRIBE
LMP_____NORMAL			
PELVIC PAIN			
ABNL VAGINAL DISCHARGE			
OTHER PROBLEMS			
LAB REVIEWED			
SLIDES REVIEWED			
SEEING COUNSELOR			

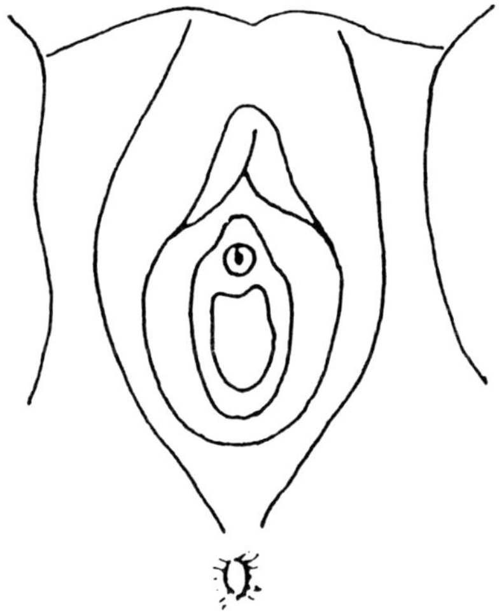

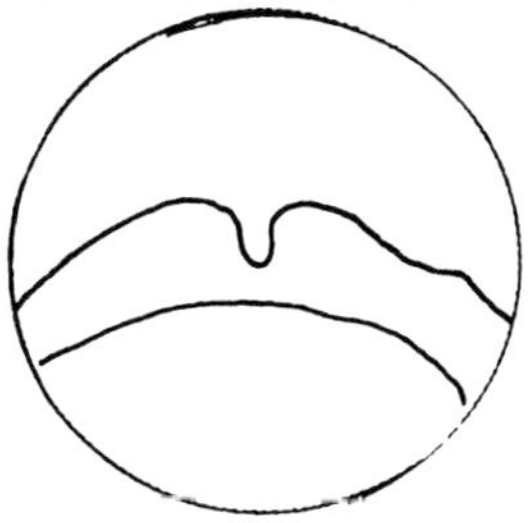

ORAL

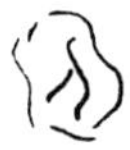

ANAL

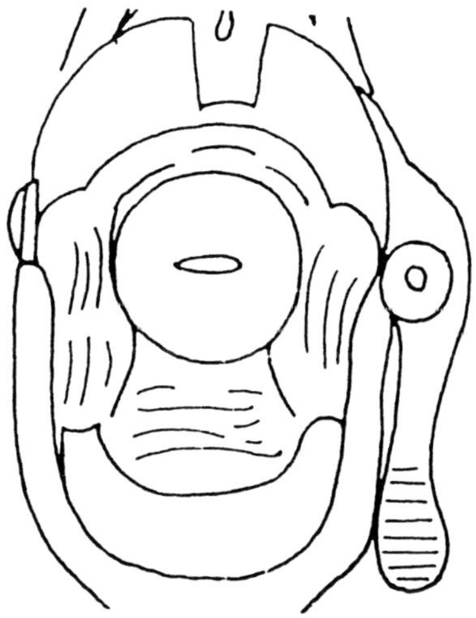

LAB:	YES	NO
CHLAMYDIA		
GC		
RPR		
HIV		
SHCG		
OTHER		
COLPO/35MM		

SUMMARY	YES	NO
COMPLETE RESOLUTION		
RESIDUAL TRAUMA		
RESIDUAL (NON/GENITAL) TRAUMA		
NEW FINDINGS		

TX/RECOMMENDATIONS _____

EXAMINER: _____

3/96   ANUS / RECTAL EXAMINATION

                                                    YES   NO

1. Anus External Examination

                            A. Injuries   ___   ___

                            B. Toluidine Dye Used ___   ___

                            C. Swabs   ___   ___

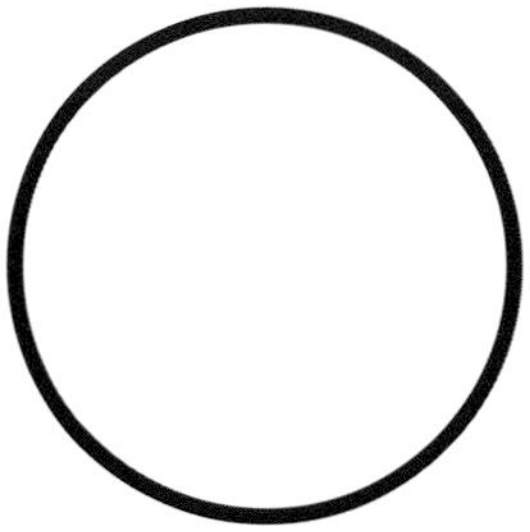

2. Anus Proximal Internal Examination
    (0.5 to 3 cm)   A. Injuries   ___   ___

                            B. Swabs   ___   ___

                            C. Lubricant   ___   ___

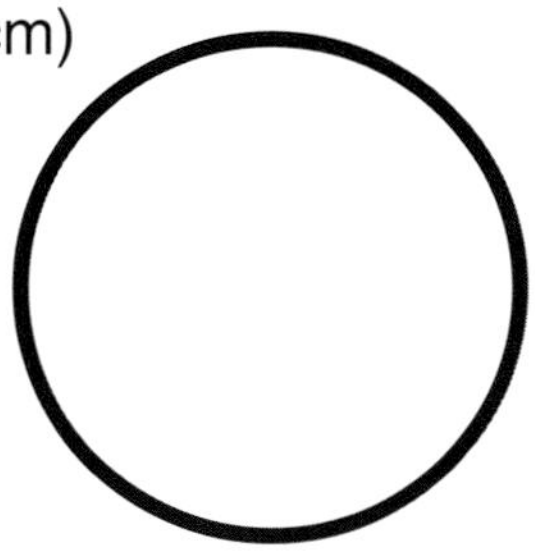

3. Rectal Distal Internal Examination
    (3 to 5 cm)   A. Injuries   ___   ___

                            B. Swabs   ___   ___

                            C. Lubricant   ___   ___

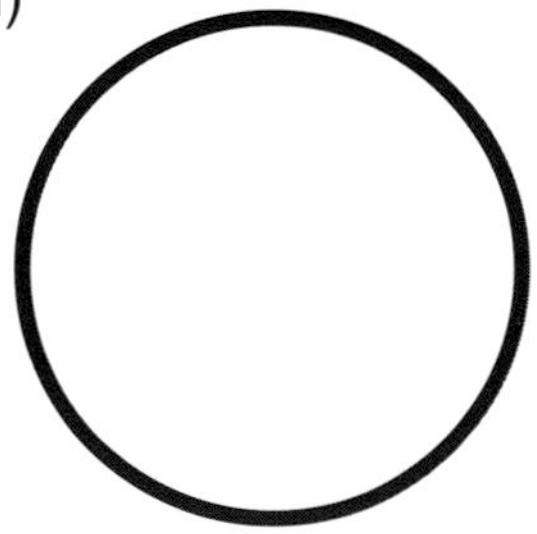

Comments: _____

_____

_____

_____

RN: _____ Date: _____

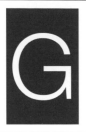

RESOURCES FOR THE EXAMINER*

American Academy of Forensic Sciences (AAFS)
P.O. Box 669
Colorado Springs, CO 80901
(719) 636-1100
e-mail: membership@aafs.org
URL: www.aafs.org

AAFS is a membership organization that provides information about careers and educational programs concerning forensics. They sponsor a annual forensic science conference.

American Society of Forensic Odontology
239 Pearl Street
Burlington, VT 05401
(802) 864-5315
FAX: (802) 864-5315
Manual available from **e-mail:** skrivera@global 2000.net

American Society for Testing Materials (ASTM)
100 Barr Harbor Drive
West Conshohocken, PA 19428-2959
(610) 832-9500
e-mail: service@astm.org

This organization has a Committee on Forensic Science for the purpose of promoting knowledge and the development of standards relating to forensic science. Subcommittees include Criminalistics, Jurisprudence, Odontology, Physical Anthropology, and Toxicology, among others.

Bureau of Justice Statistics Clearinghouse
U.S. Department of Justice
P.O. Box 179
Annapolis Junction, MD 20701-0179
(800) 732-3277
URL: ncjrs.aspensys.com:81/ncjrshome.html
or the *Statistics* section of the Department of Justice gopher at URL: www.ojp.usdoj.gov/bjs

The Clearinghouse publishes reports on various crime statistics.

Federal Bureau of Investigation
U.S. Department of Justice
Washington, DC 20535
The FBI publishes *Uniform Crime Reports for the United States,* for sale by the Superintendent of Documents, U.S. Government Printing Office, Washington, DC 20402

*A listing of courses in the United States, Canada, and Europe which prepare the sexual assault examiner and programs leading to a master's degree in Forensic Nursing may be obtained from the IAFN. A listing of undergraduate and graduate degree programs in Forensic Science is available through AAFS. Courses such as bite marks, criminal justice, fingerprinting, forensic photography, forensic science, and profiling perpetrators are also available through various sources.

International Association of Forensic Nurses (IAFN)
6900 Grove Road
Thorofare, NJ 08086
(609) 848-8356
e-mail: iafn@slackinc.com
IAFN is a professional organization of registered nurses formed to develop, promote, and disseminate information about the science of forensic nursing.

Sexual Assault Examination: Essential Forensic Techniques {video}
With a training manual: $295; available through *Western Nurse Specialists,* A Business Center Drive; Redlands, CA 92373; (909) 796-6300, 1 FAX: (909) 796-3007; **e-mail:** wns@earthlink.net

U.S. Department of Commerce
Economics and Statistics Administration
Washington, DC 20531
The Department of Commerce publishes the *Statistical Abstract of the United States,* an extensive resource for crime statistics.

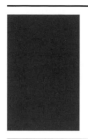

GLOSSARY

abrasion A scraping away of a portion of skin or mucous membrane, resulting when the skin contacts a rough object with sufficient force

adnexa Pelvic appendages adjacent to the uterus, usually including the fallopian tubes and ovaries

adolescence Period from beginning of puberty until sexual maturity; used here as 13 through 17 years

adult The sexually mature individual; those 18 years and older

advocate A person who aligns themselves with the patient, providing emotional support, contact with social services, arrangements for transportation, presence in court, and for other needs

alleged Asserted before proving; typically used in a legal sense

alternative light source 450 nanometer (nm) visible blue light; when this light illuminates the skin, there may be an augmentation in the appearance of pattern injuries when viewed through colored blocking filters (Golden, 1994)

anal canal Terminal portion of the large bowel, extending from the rectum at the dentate line to the anus

anal dilatation Immediate opening (within 30 seconds) of the external and internal anal sphincters with minimal traction on the buttocks

anal fissure A superficial break or split in the perianal skin, which radiates out from the anal orifice

anal fold flattening A reduction or absence of the anal folds; occurs normally when the external anal sphincter is partially or completely relaxed

anal folds See perianal folds

anal laxity Decrease in muscle tone of the anal sphincter, resulting in dilatation of the anus

anorectal line The line where the rectal columns interconnect with the anal papilla; also called dentate line

anal skin tag A protrusion of perianal tissue that interrupts the symmetry of the perianal skin folds; does not smooth out with traction

anal spasm An involuntary contraction of the anal sphincter muscles; may be attended by pain and interference with function

anal venous congestion Pooling of venous blood in the perianal tissues resulting in a purple discoloration, which may be localized or diffuse

anger rapist

- The sexual behavior is an expression of anger and rage.
- Sexuality serves an aggressive aim with the victim representing a hated person or persons from whom the rapist has experienced or has imagined insults.
- The rapist is a misogynist.

anus The anal orifice; the outlet of the large bowel

arraignment First court appearance; the defendant may plead *guilty, not guilty,* or *no contest*

bacterial vaginosis A condition in which the lactobacillus of the vagina are replaced with high concentrations of anaerobic bacteria, *Gardnerella vaginalis*, and mycoplasma hominis; symptoms are vaginal discharge and malodor

bindle A sheet of paper, folded in such a way as to contain evidence in a secure manner (see Figure 4-4 for a diagram)

bull's eye injury A patterned injury assuming the shape of the offending object; whether circular, oval, or rectangle, there is a pale center with a hypervascular or petechial surrounding area

cervical os Opening in the cervix leading into the uterine cavity

cervicitis Inflammation of the cervix

cervix The neck of the uterus, penetrated by the cervical canal; it is about 2.5 cm in length, with a rounded surface that protrudes into the vagina; for descriptive purposes the rounded surface is divided in half at the cervical os, into the anterior and posterior cervical lips

chain of custody A continuous succession of persons responsible for the evidence with the purpose to ensure there is no alteration nor loss of evidence; the documentation of the chain of custody is a record of times, places, and personnel who have been responsible for the evidence; transfers should be kept to a minimum; all transfers of custody of evidence must be logged with the (1) name of the person transferring custody (2) name of person receiving custody, and (3) date and time of the transfer; the documentation may be attached to the evidence envelope

chlamydia trachomatis An organism resembling bacteria that causes nongonococcal urethritis and pelvic inflammatory disease (PID)

clitoris Erectile tissues structurally analogous to a male penis located beneath the mons pubis, between the labia, and above the urethra; the clitoris is covered by the clitoral hood or prepuce

colposcope An instrument with a magnifying lens; it provides binocular vision, with various magnifications and the ability to take photographs; 15 times magnification is commonly used, but the possible range is 5 times to 30 times; the photographic record of the genital area is useful for consulting and as court evidence; it supports the physical findings; video camera recording may also be a feature; colposcopy magnification improves the identification of microscopic injury from 10% to 30% without colposcopy to 87% with colposcopy (Slaughter, Brown, 1992); handheld magnifiers without camera are used by some to detect microinjury

condylomata acuminata Genital or perianal warts caused by the human papilloma virus (HPV)

condylomata lata Papules of secondary syphilis

contusion An injury in which the skin is not broken; a bruise; there may be discoloration, pain, and swelling

copulation Sexual intercourse; also called coitus, concubitus; oral copulation occurs with the entry of the penis into the mouth of the victim

cunnilingus Sexual activity in which the mouth and tongue are used to stimulate the female genitalia

cut A dividing of the skin as a result of a sharp object coming against the skin with sufficient force to divide the skin; a cut is commonly confused with laceration, which is due to blunt force

cyst Fluid-filled elevation of tissue

dentate line Location where the rectal columns interconnect with the anal papilla; also called anorectal line

diastasis ani A congenital midline smooth depression that may be V-shaped or wedge-shaped and is located either anterior or posterior to the anus; a result of failure of fusion of the underlying external anal sphincter muscle

ecchymosis An irregularly formed hemorrhagic area of the skin; the color is blue-black, changing to greenish brown or yellow

ectropion Exposed columnar epithelium from the cervical canal that appears as a symmetrical circumscribed redness around the cervical os; also called eversion

elderly Typically those age 65 or older

epididymis Tube that passes from the testes to the vas deferens

erosion An alteration of the epithelium on a portion of the cervix as a result of irritation

erythema Diffused redness caused by capillary dilatation

exploitive rapist

- The sexual behavior is expressed as an impulsive predatory act. The rapist may be described as a man on the prowl for a woman to exploit sexually.
- The rapist has no concern about the experience of the victim.

fellatio Oral stimulation of the penis

felony A crime punishable by one or more of the following: fine, restitution, county jail, probation, death or other stipulation; rape is a felony

FISH Fluorescence in situ hybridization; a test that identifies male epithelial cells in semen, dried saliva, or from digital penetration by using X and Y chromosome-specific DNA probes; it is useful when there are neither spermatozoa present nor acid phosphatase elevations from the vaginal swabs; male cells may be demonstrated even 3 weeks postassault, if not contaminated from subsequent intercourse (Rao and others, 1995)

fornix, vaginal Anterior and posterior spaces in which the upper vagina is divided; the spaces are formed by the protrusion of the cervix into the vagina

fossa navicularis Concavity anterior to the posterior fourchette and posterior to the hymen

gardnerella vaginalis Pathologic bacteria; sexually transmitted; formerly called hemophilus vaginalis

genital warts Also called venereal warts and condylomata acuminata; caused by human papilloma virus (HPV)

genitalia (external) Also called the vulva; in females, it includes the mons pubis, labia majora, labia minora, clitoris, and vestibule of the vagina; the vestibule contains the urinary meatus, vaginal opening, and vestibular gland ducts

gonorrhea Infection by gram-negative diplococci *Neisseria gonorrhea* of the urethra, cervix, rectum, pharynx, or eyes; may evolve into bacteremia

hearing A legal proceeding that determines whether there is sufficient evidence for the defendant to stand trial as charged

hemorrhoid A mass of dilated, tortuous veins in the anorectum involving the venous plexuses of that area; external hemorrhoids are at the junction of the anal mucosa and anal skin; internal hemorrhoids are at the anorectal line

hepatitis B Caused by hepatitis B virus (HBV), which may enter by the parenteral route or be transmitted sexually; in 1981 a vaccine for use in preventing hepatitis B was licensed

herpes genitalis A viral infection of the genital and anorectal skin and mucosa with herpes virus Type 2; herpes is usually spread by sexual contact; there is itching and soreness followed by a small patch of erythema; a vesicle appears that erodes, resulting in shallow, small, painful ulcers on red bases; these heal in about 10 days.

hymen A membranous collar or semicollar that surrounds the vaginal introitus and separates the external genitalia from the vagina; the outer surface is squamous epithelium and the inner surface is mucous membrane; all females have this structure, and there is wide anatomic variation in morphology:

Annular (circumferential) The hymenal membrane extends completely around the circumference of the vaginal opening

Crescentic Hymen with anterior attachments at approximately the 11 o'clock and 1 o'clock position; there is no hymenal tissue at 12 o'clock

Cribriform A hymen with multiple openings

Imperforate Hymen with no opening

Microperforate Small hymenal opening

Septate The hymen has bands of tissue attached to either edge, creating two or more openings

Terms relating to the hymen

Estrogenized Effect of influence by the female sex hormone estrogen, resulting changes to the genitalia; the hymen takes on a thickened, redundant, pale appearance

Fimbriated/denticular Hymen with multiple projections along the edge creating a ruffled appearance

Redundant Abundant hymenal tissue that tends to fold back on itself or protrude

hymenal bump Solid elevation of hymenal tissue; may be seen at the site where an intravaginal ridge attaches to the hymen

hymenal cleft A nonacute transection of the hymen that does not extend to the vaginal wall; if the cleft is in the lower poles of the hymen, then it can be a healed partial transection or a congenital variation of normal; the cleft may be an angular or V-shaped indentation on the edge of the hymenal membrane or curved creating a hollowed or U-shaped depression on the edge of the membrane (*see also* hymenal transection)

hymenal notch An indentation or depression at the edge of the hymen

hymenal opening enlargement This term should be reserved for prepubertal cases in which the measurements of the horizontal or anterior-posterior diameter of the hymenal orifice are larger than two standard deviations above the mean, by age group, using published data (McCann and others, 1990)

hymenal tag Tags of tissue projecting from the rim of the hymen; these most commonly occur in the midline

hymenal transection A complete or partial tear or laceration through the width of the hymenal membrane extending to (partial) or through (complete) its attachment to the vaginal wall; if the transection is nonacute and does not extend to the vaginal wall, it is called a cleft; hymenal transections may be associated with acute and nonacute injuries (Heger, 1996)

introitus An opening or entrance into a canal or cavity as in the vaginal introitus

labia majora Outer lips to vagina; covered by pubic hair after menarche; a single lip is called the labium majus

labia minora Inner lips to vagina; in the adult, they enclose the structures of the vestibule; a single lip is called the labium minus

labial adhesion Agglutination or fusion of the labia minora in the midline; most commonly occurs posterior to hymenal orifice; can also be seen anteriorly

laceration An injury in the soft tissues resulting from ripping crushing, overstretching, pulling apart, bending, and shearing; lacerations result from blunt force and are also called tears; laceration is represented in the acronym TEARS by the *T* or *tear;* in contrast to lacerations, cuts come from sharp objects.

medical-legal examination A specialized history and physical examination performed by an examiner specializing in forensics; the purpose of the examination is to properly collect, document, and preserve evidence, as well as maintain the chain of custody; the examiner determines whether the findings support the history and timing of the event and whether there is evidence of sexual contact; standard examination guidelines are published by the American Society for Testing Materials (ASTM) (see Appendix G)

median raphe Midline fusion external from the posterior fourchette toward the anus; not a scar; also called the midline commissure

misdemeanor A crime punishable by one or more of the following: less than 1 year in a county jail, fine, probation, restitution, or other punishment

moniliasis Infection by a yeastlike fungi, chiefly *candida albicans*, causing white, cheesy discharge

mons pubis The rounded, fleshy prominence created by the underlying fat pad, which lies over the symphysis pubis (pubic bone) in the female

mounting injury Lacerations, ecchymosis, abrasions, redness, or swelling associated with the blunt force trauma of nonconsensual intromission and occurring primarily on the posterior fourchette, labia minora, hymen, and fossa navicularis from 3 o'clock to 9 o'clock; these injuries may be similar to accidental straddle injuries

nabothian cysts Retention cysts formed by an occlusion of the mouth of the nabothian glands on the cervix; may follow cervicitis

neovascularization New blood vessel formation in abnormal tissue or in an abnormal location

o'clock designation A method by which the location of structures or findings may be identified by using the numerals on the face of a clock; the 12 o'clock position is always superior; the 6 o'clock position is always inferior; identify the position of the patient when using this description

penetration Process of entering within a part; the legal definition varies by jurisdiction; in one jurisdiction, the legal definition is entering, however slight, a genital or anal opening by a penis, foreign object, or body part; the definition of oral copulation and masturbation require contact only (Office of Criminal Justice Planning, 1987)

penis Male sex organ composed of erectile tissue through which the urethra passes; composed of the shaft and glans; the glans may be covered by foreskin

perianal folds Wrinkles or folds radiating from the anus, which are created by contraction of the external anal sphincter; also called perianal folds

perianal venous congestion The collection of venous blood in the perianal tissues creating a *flat* purple discoloration; may be localized or diffuse

perianal venous engorgement Pooling of venous blood in the perianal tissues creating a bluish-purple *bulging* of the tissues; may be localized or diffuse

perineum The external surface of the perineal body, lying between the posterior fourchette and anus in females and the scrotum and anus in males

periurethral support bands Small bands lateral to the urethra that connect the periurethral tissue to the wall of the vestibule; these normal supportive structures are also called vestibular bands and support bands

perpetrator classification The four main types of rapists classified according to studies of descriptions of convicted rapists and the interaction of sexual and aggressive motivations; the four types are (1) anger rapist (2.5%), (2) exploitive rapist (5%), (3) power reassurance rapist (90%), (4) sadistic rapist (2.5%) (Douglas and others, 1992; Ressler, 1992)

petechiae Small purplish, hemorrhagic spots on the skin or mucous membranes; may be singular or multiple

posterior fornix Vaginal cavity located beneath the cervix

posterior fourchette A tense band or fold of mucous membrane at the posterior commissure of the vagina, connecting the posterior ends of the labia minora; in the prepubertal child, this area is referred to as a posterior commissure because the labia minora are not completely developed to connect posteriorly until puberty; the fossa navicularis is the culdesac anterior to the fourchette and that which separates the fourchette from the hymen

power-reassurance rapist

- The assault is primarily an expression of rape fantasies. The rapist fantasizes that the victim will enjoy the experience.
- There is typically a history of sexual preoccupation with a variety of perversions, including bizarre masturbatory practices, voyeurism, exhibitionism, obscene telephone calls, cross dressing, and fetishisms.
- There is a distorted perception of the victim/offender relationship. The rapist may want the victim to respond in a sexual or erotic manner and may even try to make a date after the assault.
- This is an individual who is compensating for his acutely felt inadequacies as a male.

proctitis Inflammation of the rectum

prostate Gland that produces semen

rape The legal definition varies from state to state, but typically includes three criteria: (1) unwillingness to engage in an act, (2) force or coercion, or (3) mental or physical inability to communicate; the crime of rape requires only slight penile penetration; full erection and ejaculation is not necessary; rape occurs to males and females (Bureau of Justice Statistics, 1995; Burgess, and others, 1995), between married persons, and persons of the same gender; rape is a form of sexual assault

rectum Lower part of the large intestine, between sigmoid flexure and anal canal; separated from the anal canal at the dentate line

sadistic rapist

- There is a fusion between sexual and aggressive feelings. As sexual arousal increases, aggressive

feelings increase, and as aggression increases, sexual arousal increases as well.

- The anger may begin to emerge as the offender becomes sexually aroused. This results in bizarre and intense forms of sexual-aggressive violence against parts of the body having sexual significance such as the breasts, anus, buttocks, genitals, and mouth.

scar Fibrous tissue that replaces normal tissue after the healing of a wound; as in an episiotomy scar

sentence Penalty pronounced by the judge, based on testimony, arguments, legal requirements, precedence, and probation department recommendations; there are often substantial differences in the penalty for like offenses

sexual assault Definition varies by state; in California (1990), sexual assault is: (1) force, threats, or coercion to engage in an unwanted sexual act; (2) contact or penetration of the intimate parts (sexual organs, anus, groin, buttocks, and breasts) of one person with another person; included is rape, rape with a foreign object, rape by a spouse, forced oral copulation, forced sodomy, attempted rape, and sexual battery

sexual coercion Incidents in which one person dominates another by force or compels the other person to perform a sexual act

sodomy Acts of anal penetration

survivor A term used most commonly by counselors to indicate that the sexually assaulted patient has attained a certain stage of emotional recovery

synechiae Any adhesion that binds two anatomic structures through the formation of a band of tissue; a synechia can result in the healing process following an abrasion of tissues

syphilis Disease caused by the spirochete *treponema pallidium*; characterized by sequential stages and years of latency; may affect any tissue; initial lesion appears as a red papule changing to a painless ulcer (chancre); the papules of secondary syphilis (condylomata) must be differentiated from condylomata acuminata

Tanner stages Classification to categorize secondary sexual development; the degree of sexual maturity defined by physical evidence of breast development and pubic hair in the female; the testicular, scrotal, and penile size, along with the location of pubic hair, are used in the male; range from Stage 1 (prepubertal child) to Stage 5 (fully mature adult) (Tanner, 1962);

see Chapter 4 for diagrams of the sexual development of females and males

TEARS acronym

T   Tear (laceration) or tenderness
E   Ecchymosis (bruise)
A   Abrasion
R   Redness (erythema)
S   Swelling (edema)

tear/laceration An injury in the soft tissues, resulting from ripping, crushing, overstretching, pulling apart, bending, and shearing; lacerations result from blunt force; in contrast, cuts come from sharp objects.

ecchymosis Irregular hemorrhagic areas of the skin; the color is blue-black changing to greenish brown or yellow; it is caused from extravasation of blood into skin or mucous membrane

abrasion A scraping away of a portion of skin or mucous membrane from injury or mechanical means

redness/erythema A form of macula with diffused redness, caused by capillary congestion

swelling A local or general accumulation of fluids in the tissues

testes Male sex organs that produce spermatozoa

Toluidine Blue dye 1% aqueous solution dyes nucleated squamous cells in the deeper layers of the epidermis exposed by lacerations; deep blue uptake is interpreted as positive for injury; inflammatory causes, as well as benign or malignant vulvovaginal disease permit dye uptake but in a diffuse pattern (Lauber, Souma, 1982); Toluidine Blue dye is effective in dark-skinned people and does not highlight episiotomy scars (McCauley and others, 1987); gloves and eye protection should be worn during use (Spectrum Chemical Manufacturing Corporation, 1991) (see Chapter 4)

trial By judge or by jury where all evidence, information, and testimony is presented; it is followed by a judgment of guilt or innocence and if guilty, a sentence

trichomoniasis A single-celled protozoan; sexually transmitted and causes burning and itching of vulva with yellow-green discharge; most males are asymptomatic carriers

urethra Opening to the bladder

uterus Reproductive organ composed of a cervix, corpus, and fundus

vagina Tubular structure with convoluted rugae that stretch anatomically from the hymen to the cervix; the vaginal rugae account in part for the ability of the vagina to distend

vaginitis Inflammation of the vagina resulting from infection or postmenopausal (senile or atrophic) changes; atrophic vaginitis is characterized by discharge, burning and soreness; there may be asymmetrical redness around the cervix and friable tissues that bleed with little or no trauma; local estrogen is used for treatment; in contrast, normal vaginal atrophy occurs with decreasing estrogen and is noninflammatory

vas deferens Tube from epididymis to the urethra

venereal warts Condyloma acuminatum; warty lesions on the labia and within the vestibule

venous lakes Purplish discoloration of the skin; lakes become more prominent with separation and disappear as traction is released

vestibular bands Symmetrical bands lateral to the urethra (periurethral bands) or hymen (perihymenal bands) and connect to the vestibular wall

vestibular papillae Small elevations that are grouped and appear in the area of the vestibule; the papillae occur as a result of hormonally triggered changes that occur in minor vestibular glands at the transitional epithelium; papillae are most typical in adolescents

vestibule of vagina An almond-shaped space between the lines of attachment of the labia minora; four structures open into the vestibule—urethral orifice, vaginal orifice, and two ducts of the glands of Bartholin

vulva The portion of the female external genitalia consisting of the labia majora, labia minora, clitoris, vaginal vestibule (urethral orifice, vaginal orifice, Bartholin ducts), hymen, fossa navicularis, and posterior fourchette

vulvitis Inflammation of the vulva

Woods' lamp Ultraviolet light; a component of the invisible spectrum of light; it is capable of fluorescing semen, some detergents, and certain clothing fibers; best used in a darkened room

REFERENCES

Barkow R, editor: *The Merck manual of diagnosis and therapy,* ed 16, Rathway, NJ 1992, Merck.

Burgess AW and others: Victim care services and the comprehensive sexual assault assessment tool. In Hazelwood R, Burgess AW, editors: *Practical aspects of rape investigation,* ed 2, 1995, CRC Press.

Bureau of Justice Statistics: *Violence against women: estimates from the redesigned survey,* Washington, DC, 1995, U.S. Department of Justice.

California Attorney General: *Women's rights handbook,* Sacramento, Calif, 1990, Author.

Centers for Disease Control and Prevention: Sexually transmitted diseases treatment guidelines, *MMWR* 42, No RR-14, 1993, US Department of Health and Human Services.

Committee on Terminology: Descriptive terminology in child sexual abuse medical evaluations, *Practice guideline,* 1995, American Professional Society on the Abuse of Children.

Council on Scientific Affairs, American Medical Association. Violence against women: relevance for medical practitioners, *J Am Med Assn* 276:3184, 1992.

Douglas JE and others: *Crime classification manual* New York, 1992, Lexington.

Golden G: Use of alternative light source illumination in bite mark photography, *J Foren Sci* 39:815, 1994.

Heger, A: Personal communication, November 1996.

Lauber AA, Souma ML: Use of Toluidine Blue for documentation of traumatic intercourse, *Ob Gyn* 60:622, 1982.

McCann and others: Genital findings in prepubertal girls selected for non-abuse: a descriptive study, *Pediatr* 86:428, 1990.

McCauley J and others: Toluidine blue in the corroboration of rape in the adult victim, *Am J Emerg Med* 2:105, 1987.

Office in Criminal Justice Planning: *California medical protocol for examination of sexual assault and child sexual abuse victims,* Sacramento, Calif, 1987, Author.

Rao P and others: Identification of male epithelial cells in routine post coital cervicovaginal smears using fluorescence in situ hybridization, *Am J Clin Pathol* 104:32, 1995.

Slaughter L, Brown CRV: Colposcopy to establish physical findings in rape victims, *Am J OB Gyn* 166:83, 1992.

Spectrum Chemical Manufacturing Corporation: *Toluidine Blue 1% as used in sexual assault: spectrum characteristics,* specifications revised, 1991; FAX:310-516-9843.

Stedman's Concise Medical Dictionary, ed 2, Baltimore, 1994, Williams and Wilkins.

Tanner JM: *Growth at adolescence,* ed 2, Oxford, 1962, Blackwell Scientific.

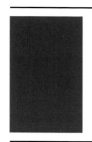

INDEX